your guide to
back pain

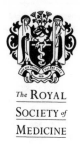

The ROYAL
SOCIETY *of*
MEDICINE

your guide to
back pain

Dr John Tanner

MBBS, DM-SM, DSMSA
Registered Osteopath

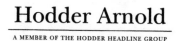

Hodder Arnold

A MEMBER OF THE HODDER HEADLINE GROUP

Hodder Arnold have agreed to pay 50 pence per product
on all sales made of this title to the retailer at a discount of
up to and including 60% from the UK Recommended
Retail Price to BackCare.

Orders: Please contact Bookpoint Ltd, 130 Milton Park,
Abingdon, Oxon OX14 4SB. Telephone: (44) 01235 827720,
Fax: (44) 01235 400454. Lines are open from 9.00 to
18.00, Monday to Saturday, with a 24-hour message
answering service. You can also order through our website
www.hoddereducation.com

British Library Cataloguing in Publication Data
A catalogue record for this title is available from the British
Library.

ISBN-10: 0 340 90499 2
ISBN-13: 9 780340 904992

First published   2005
Impression number   10 9 8 7 6 5 4 3 2 1
Year   2008   2007   2006   2005

Typeset by Servis Filmsetting Limited, Longsight, Manchester.
Printed in Great Britain for Hodder Arnold, a division of
Hodder Headline, 338 Euston Road, London NW1 3BH,
by Cox & Wyman Ltd, Reading, Berkshire.

Hodder Headline's policy is to use papers that are natural,
renewable and recyclable products and made from wood
grown in sustainable forests. The logging and manufacturing
processes are expected to conform to the environmental
regulations of the country of origin.

Every effort has been made to trace copyright for material used
in this book. The authors and publishers would be happy to
make arrangements with any holder of copyright whom it has
not been possible to trace successfully by the time of going to
press.

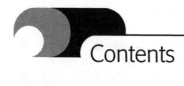

Contents

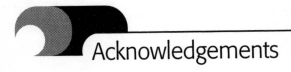

Acknowledgements

I would like to thank Jenny Meltzer for typing up the manuscript, Dr Peter Skew for his helpful comments, numerous patients whose experiences and stories I have drawn from and whom have been my greatest teachers and my own family for their forbearance while I have been busy with this book.

Yours

John

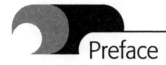

Preface

This new book, published in partnership with the Royal Society of Medicine, provides detailed, useful and up-to-date information on back pain. It contains expert yet user-friendly advice, with such useful features as:

Key Terms: demystifying the jargon
Questions and Answers: answering the burning questions
Myths and Facts: debunking the misconceptions
My Experience: how it feels to live with, or care for someone with, this condition.

Bearing the hallmark of excellence and accessibility that characterizes the work of the Royal Society of Medicine, this important guide will enable you and your family to gain some control over the way your back pain is managed by being better informed.

Peter Richardson
Director of Publications
Royal Society of Medicine

Introduction

Back pain has been with us throughout our evolutionary history and will probably remain so for the foreseeable future. This book is an attempt to increase the reader's understanding of the many manifestations of pain arising from the spine and the ways in which it can be managed by the doctor and therapist as well as the reader himself. It is designed to bring hope to those who feel that their personal experience with back pain has not been adequately recognised or too readily dismissed.

I believe that it has come at a timely moment when health services for musculoskeletal pain are being revised in favour of a new and radically different strategy for delivery of care. These changes will hopefully enable the sufferer to receive good care and advice at the primary care level, supported by interface clinics, based largely in the community rather than in hospitals, with doctors and therapists specifically trained in the diagnosis and treatment of spinal pain and other musculoskeletal disorders.

xii   your guide to back pain

The consequence is not, of course, freedom for all from back pain but it should at least reduce the burden of chronic back pain and disability on society and the individual, allowing many more people to lead fulfilling lives in employment and recreation.

CHAPTER

1

Why me?

'Why me?' is a question that most people ask at some point when they are struck by an acute episode of back pain. Half of all such occurrences appear to come on without any obvious preceding warning or causative factor. If you mentally rewind the previous day's or few days' activity you may recall some awkward twisting motion or action that may have strained something. You may have felt a momentary glitch or twang in the back which at the time did not seem particularly significant. On the other hand, you may be used to doing these sorts of activities on a regular basis and cannot understand why your back is acting up this time.

In the other half of such cases, there is an obvious trigger such as some heavy lifting strain, moving some furniture in your house or putting something heavy in the back of your car. Sometimes there is simply an ache or a few twinges which build up over a few hours, and the next morning the severe pain comes on when you try to get out of bed. **Epidemiology**

epidemiology
The study of illness, disease and disorders in society.

informs us about the common ailment of back pain.

Up to 80 per cent of the population experiences back trouble at some time in their lives. Surveys tell us that up to 50 per cent of the population will have experienced some discomfort or pain in their back in the preceding year. This is called the 'prevalence' of back pain, and the results of these surveys tell us that back pain is basically very common (see Figure 1.1 below).

In fact, one might almost call back pain a natural condition of humankind. The peak incidence of onset of significant back pain is between the ages of 30 and 50, although as many as 15 per cent of children and adolescents also experience backache of the common and garden variety. Putting it into perspective, however severe the pain might be, you are experiencing something that occurs commonly to people at some time in their lives. People can often assume that as the pain is so severe, it means that there is something seriously wrong.

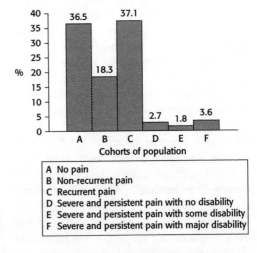

A No pain
B Non-recurrent pain
C Recurrent pain
D Severe and persistent pain with no disability
E Severe and persistent pain with some disability
F Severe and persistent pain with major disability

Figure 1.1 Prevalence of back pain one year after an acute episode (Von Korff, Spine Journal, 1991).

It should be reassuring to state at this stage that the incidence of serious back pain caused by disease or pathology is actually less than 1 per cent. In other words, there is a very high chance that you are suffering from one of the many causes of common back pain. The self-diagnosis chart in the Appendix will help you to sort through your symptom picture to reach a working self-diagnosis.

> **myth**
> The pain in my back is so severe it must mean there's something seriously wrong.

> **fact**
> Only 1 per cent of back pain is due to serious disease or pathology.

Vulnerability to back pain

Physical and health factors

Women are a little more vulnerable to back pain than men, possibly due to the influence of pregnancy, childbirth and bringing up a child, all of which can take their toll.

It seems logical that posture and how the back is used on a daily basis have some effect on producing or preventing back pain. However, there is little evidence for this, although later chapters will explain that attention to posture and optimal use of the spine can clearly influence recovery and reduce symptoms. It also seems logical that fitness and strength might help protect someone from back pain but, once again there is not much evidence in favour of this. The main evidence for fitness and strength comes in prevention of recurrent attacks or reducing the impact of chronic back pain. Tall people are more vulnerable, due to the leverage on their lower spine but, surprisingly enough, obese people are not significantly more likely to develop first-time back pain. There is increasing evidence that people whose arteries are becoming blocked with atheromatous (fatty) deposits, or those on a poor diet who smoke will be more likely to have degeneration of the spinal **discs**. This may in turn lead to an increased chance of back pain.

> **discs**
> The matrix of fibre and cartilage sandwiched between the vertebrae.

Employment factors

Epidemiological studies on the incidence and prevalence of back trouble in the workforce do suggest a relationship between the amount of heavy work done and the likelihood of getting back trouble. Heavy manual workers are more likely to take time off work due to back pain, and this may of course include nurses as much as heavy construction workers. However, the prevalence of back pain in modern society is so high that even sedentary workers are experiencing nearly the same degree of risk (see Figure 1.2).

Workers involved in the intermediate 'moderate' category such as packers, retail workers and agricultural workers will all report a significant amount of back pain, which may lead to time off work. Recent research suggests that the cause of these relatively high incidences of reporting of back pain and loss of time from work are not so much related to the actual loads experienced by the spine or ergonomic factors at work, but to more subtle issues such as the way sickness absence is managed in the workplace, and employment legislation.

Q Is this new pain due to the work I do?

A Not necessarily. There are many factors that contribute towards back pain and studies suggest that the kind of work a person does plays only a small part. However, heavy manual workers are more likely to take sick leave due to back pain than other members of the workforce.

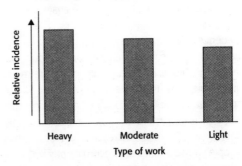

| **Figure 1.2** Back pain at work.

Protecting the worker encourages immediate reporting of incidents and may involve the health and safety officer and the worker's union. The question of who is to blame often arises.

myth
Having a bad back means I shall never be able to do my proper work. I will have to retire or change my job.

fact
One of the biggest risk factors for developing chronic pain is low job satisfaction. Stress, unhappiness at work with colleagues or work supervisor, and a feeling of loss of control or autonomy over one's own working environment are all poor motivating factors and tend to lead to prolonged work absence and perpetuation of symptoms and disability.

In the present risk-averse culture, if a person develops back pain at work, whether they tripped over a carpet or stumbled down the steps, the employer is potentially liable. This can lead to a vicious circle whereby the pain and disability experienced by the injured worker become a lever to obtain injury compensation. This escalates when people in authority must be convinced that the pain is genuine – documentation must be sought and treatment and investigations pursued, leading to prolongation of the time to recovery. Furthermore, employers and public services are required to protect themselves by making sure that their employee does not return to work carrying a current injury which may be aggravated by work, therefore insisting that the person is 100 per cent fit before returning to full employment. Of course the assumption underlying this is that the person was 100 per cent fit before the onset of back pain, which is extremely unlikely.

The important point to note is that this process does not always lead to the quickest route to health and recovery. There may of course be genuine negligence where a particular task imposes unreasonable loads or a working environment is inherently unsafe or an accident is simply 'waiting to happen', but these circumstances are relatively rare. Most back pain at work occurs in much the same way as it occurs at home or on the sports field – by an awkward bend, twist or stumble.

A different perspective

Looking at in another way, the concern may actually lie in being able to get back to a favourite sport or recreation as fast as possible. The injured sportsperson or athlete is highly motivated to get fit in order to play with their team or progress in their sporting career. Downtime is minimized and active rehabilitation sought, with the sportsperson taking full responsibility in most situations for the strain or overstrain which occurred and the need to get the balance of training and competition right.

What causes back pain?

In the past, X-rays were frequently ordered to locate the cause of back pain. Most of the time they will show nothing that increases understanding of the cause of the problem, however, sometimes irrelevant abnormalities show up. These commonly include the following:

✧ Mild 'scoliosis', meaning a rotation curvature of the spine which is fairly common to a mild degree. Severe curvature (more than 45 degrees) is very noticeable and does need special medical attention

✧ An excessive convexity, called 'kyphosis', affects posture but is really most significant in the sporting adolescent involved in certain activities such as gymnastics and swimming where the condition may influence the range of shoulder movement.

Other abnormalities such as **transitional vertebrae** (see Chapter 4, page 71), which alter the bony structure of the spine, occur in up to 5 per cent of the whole population and from a recent study appear to be more common in back pain sufferers.

transitional vertebrae
An abnormal development of the vertebra structure and/or its joints.

myth
If I have back pain at my age (implying young or too young), this must be a sign of a 'weak back'.

fact
At the time when you have acute disabling back pain, your back may well feel weak – sometimes your leg gives way and you cannot support your weight – but this is usually a passing phenomenon. In a few days the muscles will calm down and, through gentle movement, you will regain your strength and posture.

Most commonly, some **wear and tear** in the spine shows up as narrowing of the disc or, in older age groups, '**spondylosis**' (see Plate 1) This simply refers to the normal age-related changes of the spine which are found with increasing frequency the older you are. Some people do have a narrow spinal canal (**spinal stenosis**), which will cause more severe and more prolonged back trouble if they develop a disc prolapse. This seems to be a problem that starts very early in life and may be related to nutrition and growth as a foetus. However, it seems that all that can be done with this knowledge is to advise the individual about the consequences of heavy lifting and twisting.

wear and tear
The preferred term for all the medical labels used to describe structural changes that occur with age and use (for example, spondylosis, degeneration, osteoarthritis).

spondylosis
The changes of the margins of the vertebra due to ageing.

Q **My chiropractor says I have a scoliosis which needs long-term treatment – is this true?**

A No. If the curvature is only mild it is probably not a significant factor. If you have a true structural scoliosis, it cannot be altered through manual treatment.

spinal stenosis
An excessive narrowing of the spinal canal.

Q **Why have I suddenly experienced back pain when I haven't done anything to trigger it?**

A It is likely that your back has been subject to ageing and wear and tear over a very long period of time. This gradual process means that one day (even without a particular trigger), you will suddenly experience pain which is the culmination of years of strain.

How do back injuries occur?

When you rewind the previous day's or days' activities, you will probably remember that you worked a little too long in the attic, crouching in a corner, putting in insulation, or doing that awkward plumbing job under the sink. Prolonged bending with twisting is probably one of the most common causes of acute back pain. These tasks, together with heavy awkward lifts such as putting a roll of carpet into the back of a lorry, are some of the most frequent precipitants for acute onset of back pain. You may ask, 'Why has it happened at this particular moment?' It is probable that the spine has been silently undergoing a process of change – a combination of ageing and wear and tear – to put it in a condition where a little additional strain or overuse has been sufficient to set off an acute back strain. This may be on a par with an old rope that has been gradually fraying, with individual strands giving way silently until it is the last straw which causes the structure to give way. In other words, what you were doing yesterday or the previous day is simply the visible tip of the iceberg. The stored accumulation of wear and tear, use and misuse of the spine over two, three or four decades represents the nine-tenths of the iceberg beneath the surface.

What is meant by wear and tear?

'Wear and tear' does not necessarily refer to heavy overload or overuse, such as a gardener or road digger may incur through their job. It refers to how we use our backs on a day-to-day basis: everyday posture in the car, at home in the armchair or sofa, or doing simple chores in the house and garden. The habits that we develop in childhood, when we often chose to ignore our teachers' or parents' admonitions about our bad posture, may be beginning to tell. Weak back muscles and weak abdominal muscles may make your spine more vulnerable to overstrain. We have already referred to cardiovascular health in terms of artery blockage, and smoking and overeating, particularly fatty food, may all play a part. Unfortunately, there is no simple answer to the onset of what is commonly referred to in medical terms as 'simple backache'. The reasons for the onset of your back pain are complex and **multifactorial**.

multifactorial
Indicates that the cause of a particular condition has many sources and influences.

Q My father had a bad back all his life, is it in my genes?

A Recent studies in England and Finland show that genetic factors do play a significant role. Collagen, the protein strands in your discs and ligaments, is coded by certain genes and there is no doubt that some people make 'inferior' collagen. This accounts for up to 60 per cent of disc degeneration as shown in the studies of twins over a lifetime. Since this fact of inheritance is entirely beyond our control, it is even more important that you work on the factors that you can control.

What does the future hold?

Once you have had your first attack of back pain, the odds are you will experience a further episode – about 50–60 per cent risk within the next year or two – and this is also true for neck pain. In fact, the **natural history** of back pain shows an increasing frequency of episodes, sometimes one blending into the next over the middle decades of life, and a tendency for the severity and impact of these episodes to subside over the last two decades of life.

natural history
The course a disease or illness follows without interference from any form of medical intervention.

This does not mean that you will become crippled with disabling back pain, but it does mean that you will have to learn how to look after your back a lot better than you have been doing and not taking the health of your spine for granted. A practitioner who specializes in back pain, such as a physiotherapist (see Chapter 5), or any practitioner or doctor who takes a special interest in back pain, should be able to teach the basics of good back care. This includes postural training and use of the back for everyday activities. More details of the kind of self-help activities that can be done are found in Chapter 8. However, it is important to be aware of certain activities which increase the risk of provoking or worsening the current back pain. These include:

✧ Lifting heavy weights manually or suddenly
✧ Lifting an unexpectedly light weight
✧ Stooping and prolonged bending
✧ Bending, twisting and reaching
✧ Repetitive work with lighter loads
✧ Static work postures, as in driving, working on an assembly line, sewing and weaving
✧ Vibration from vehicles in driving jobs
✧ Monotony of job and low job satisfaction
✧ Unacceptably high workloads (workloads should consist of a maximum of half body weight for occasional handling and 40 per cent of body weight for continuous lifting)
✧ Rapid repetitive handling tasks
✧ Inappropriate working heights
✧ Poor seating without back rest, arm supports or swivel action
✧ Inadequate space within which to turn or move
✧ Risks factors at computer workstations.

With awareness of these factors and good advice, there is no reason why the future cannot be just as bright as the past with the occasional backache or episode of back pain. Very few people need to give up or change their job.

Working with back pain

In general, once someone has been off work for 4–12 weeks with back pain, they have a 10–40 per cent risk of still being off work after one year and, after one or two years' absence, it is unlikely that they will return to any form of work in the foreseeable future irrespective of further treatment (see Figure 1.3).

The best advice is to resume normal activity quickly and to return to work as soon as possible. This will lead to shorter periods of work loss, fewer recurrences and less work loss over the following year. This will of course depend on the commitment at your place of work to find ways of helping you return to work, perhaps on a part-time basis with restricted duties initially. The workplace culture and commitment from your employers in improving safety and providing maximum support are crucial in this regard.

myth
I should wait until my back pain is completely better before returning to work.

fact
The longer you are off work with back pain, the lower your chance of ever returning to work. Try to return to work as soon as possible, even if this means for just a couple of hours a day at first.

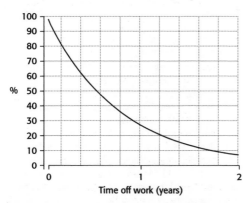

Figure 1.3 Probability of returning to work with back pain (Government Advisory Group report, 1994).

my experience

I am a 44-year-old full-time fire fighter, and I hurt my back during a training programme five years ago. I was off work for ten weeks. Two years later I had another more severe episode of back pain and it took 16 weeks to get back to work. However, this time my back never seemed to fully recover. I gave up jogging and gym workouts, gained weight and was having frequent periods of sickness absence when my back flared up again. I had been on restricted duties for a year when I was referred by an occupational health advisor to see a doctor for an independent opinion. The question was whether I should be medically retired or could any treatment return me to full fitness. After 20 years' service I would be eligible for a full pension. The service was also worried that should I have a severe attack at work, it could be sued for negligence.

I told my doctor that I felt I had given the fire service the best years of my life, my back was worn out, that I didn't think much of the way my case had been handled, and that I was initiating an injury claim on the advice of my union. All treatment had failed, I was in pain most days, particularly sitting doing office duties, and I felt that I was fully entitled to compensation since my injury occurred at work. I did feel loyal to the fire service, and didn't know what else I would do if I retired early, and I did have many friends at work. However, I said that I would consider redeployment as a trainer if that was possible, but I wanted a scan to diagnose exactly what was wrong since no one had ever been able to tell me.

The doctor examined me and diagnosed a recurrent lumbar disc syndrome and explained that having a scan would not affect management of my condition since I was not a candidate for invasive treatment (surgery).

He explained that my back problem did not necessarily result from my work since my close family had a high rate of chronic back pain and, therefore, was partly hereditary and common at my age across all occupations due to accumulated 'wear and tear'. He said that there was a risk of recurrence no matter what work I did since that was the natural history of the condition for the next 10–15 years. He explained that the best way to reduce this risk was for me to 'take responsibility 'for looking after my own back by:

1   Getting fit.
2   Losing weight.

3 Undertaking an outpatient rehabilitation programme.
4 Following a home exercise programme.

The doctor discussed the way forward with management and occupational health and supported my option for a training role for the remaining five years' service. He reassured them and me that it was unrealistic to expect 100 per cent fitness and immunity from recurrence in order to return to work in an active capacity (even as a fire fighter, since the back does not collapse during 'adrenaline moments').

CHAPTER

2

What can I do about back pain?

People vary enormously in how they cope with acute or chronic pain. It is interesting to note that a study in Sweden showed that nurses with back pain of varying severity were just as likely to continue to go to work as they were to stay at home and rest. When each case was analysed individually, there was no difference in the severity or duration of symptoms between the group of nurses who decided to stay at work and keep active and those who stayed at home. The difference seems to lie in people's attitude to pain and their ability to cope.

Other studies have shown that many people cope with pain without ever consulting a doctor or practitioner. Once again, the range of diagnoses may be similar and the severity of pain they experience from day to day is not different. The decision about what to do depends very much on the individual.

Self-help

Those people who carry on and do not seek medical help may cope with back pain by employing a number of the simple and obvious methods described on page 23. If the pain is mild or no more than a minor irritation, one option that many people choose is to ignore it and carry on with their normal activities. There is absolutely no evidence to indicate that this does any harm. In fact, there is greater evidence in support of maintaining normal activities since the natural history of back pain shows that it is a fluctuating condition which is not destined to deteriorate, providing a sensible approach is taken to the kind of activities undertaken.

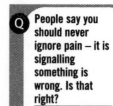

Q **People say you should never ignore pain – it is signalling something is wrong. Is that right?**

A Severe acute pain such as a spasm or violent twinge should be heeded. An aching pain that is not aggravated by normal activity often responds better to movement.

Curing back pain

Most studies over the last 20 years have successfully dispelled the traditional notion of rest being the best cure for back pain. Prolonged bed rest leads to muscle wasting, loss of fitness (**deconditioning**), **demineralization** of the bones, low mood and self-esteem, even depression in some cases and ultimately prolongs recovery time.

Many countries have produced national guidelines for managing back pain, and they all agree that prolonged rest does more harm than good. Obviously allowances should be made if the pain is so severe that it is impossible to get out of bed or move around without provoking severe painful twinges and spasms. However, this sort of pain usually subsides within two or three days of modified activity or complete rest and, as soon as possible, attempts should be made to start moving and gradually resume normal activity. To cope with more significant

deconditioning
The loss of fitness resulting from prolonged rest.

demineralization
The loss of or leaching out of minerals from your bones due to disuse.

myth
Rest is the best cure for back pain.

fact
Rest can actually lead to increasing weakness and deterioration and, in most cases, rest is not recommended.

pain, simple analgesics such as paracetamol or ibuprofen may help. There is reasonable evidence in support of non-steroidal anti-inflammatories and muscle relaxants for acute back pain but most of these, with the exception of ibuprofen, have to be prescribed by a doctor who will consider whether such medication is safe for you to use.

The use of hot or cold packs for acute pain and muscle spasms is often recommended and widely used, but of course the effects do not penetrate as far as the spine itself. However, this can be comforting in the acute phase where muscle spasm or tense muscles are part of the picture.

Modification of activity

Since back pain can come from a variety of different sources, the actual mechanics underlying the production of pain are not always easy to clarify. Therefore, over the last few decades, a variety of activity modifications have been proposed. For the lower back there is a reasonable consensus on the dos and don'ts to aid recovery from the acute phase:

✧ Try to keep your back straight, and avoid prolonged bending or leaning over
✧ Minimize sitting time or, if you must sit, keep to an upright chair with good back support for relatively short periods. Avoid soft chairs and sofas which do not give enough support
✧ Avoid heavy lifting and carrying activities until the pain and muscle tension has subsided
✧ For everyday activities such as getting out of bed and getting dressed, roll over on your side first, push up sideways from the bed, try and use your legs to stand up straight, pushing down with your arms away from the

bed. When getting dressed, avoid sitting and bending over, which increases the pressure in your lower spine. Instead, stand and bring your knee up towards you to put on socks and shoes, or lean against a wall or place your foot on a chair (see Figure 2.1) Alternatively, kneel to the floor to reach your shoes.

Q I have been advised not to do various things with a bad back, but why should I feel like an invalid at my age?

A This advice is to be followed to aid and accelerate your recovery. It will enable you to do almost everything but just in a different way. Even competitive weightlifters have to use correct techniques to look after their backs.

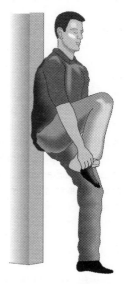

Figure 2.1 How to dress without straining your back.

The postures in Figure 2.2 on page 18 show how the pressure within the lumbar discs varies in different positions. Pressure is defined as being 100 per cent when you stand up straight.

Exercise

There is good evidence that maintaining activity and performing gentle exercise such as walking, even brisk walking, helps back pain. There is a large variety of specific therapeutic exercise programmes which are taught most often by

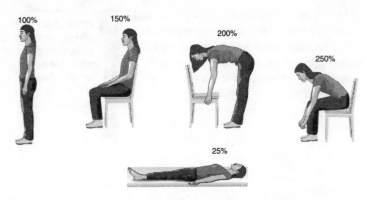

Figure 2.2 Disc pressure on the lumbar spine in different postures.

physiotherapists. The most popular regime at present is that devised by Australian physiotherapist, Robin McKenzie, which is primarily aimed at the mechanics of the disc in the lumbar spine. This regime has been popularized in McKenzie's books such as 'Treat Your Own Back,' and many people find it useful.

Self-awareness

If the pain is severe and making it difficult to move, some people quite naturally start to worry about the possible causes and implications. Some even talk in terms of feeling 'paralysed' by the pain, and this conjures up images of spinal cord injury, which is extremely rare and very unlikely to be a cause of everyday back pain. Nevertheless, these negative thoughts can start to take control, and fear and anxiety can supervene. Negative thoughts and images can escalate and if your mind turns to others you know, such as family members in the past who have been crippled by arthritis or developed cancer in the spine from a primary source such as the breast or prostate, then of course these fearful thoughts will influence how your body is reacting to the current pain. These are termed 'catastrophic thoughts' and this kind of thinking is called '**catastrophizing**'. Research by psychologists has shown that this train of thought can be one of the biggest stumbling blocks to recovery.

catastrophizing
Thinking the worst, an extreme form of pessimistic thinking.

Fear of pain is more disabling than the pain itself

Severe pain is extremely unpleasant, and it is natural to seek to avoid it. However, even severe pain can be tolerated in short bursts, and it is a fact that these pains will often subside more quickly than you realize. Yet some people start to anticipate this severe pain to the point where even a trivial movement, which is surely not harmful even though it may provoke a degree of pain, becomes a trigger for the fear. This leads to the strange situation that 'the fear of pain is more disabling than the pain itself'. This in turn leads to a behaviour termed '**fear avoidance**', which means you are avoiding doing a movement or activity for fear of the pain it might cause. This is commonly seen in some sufferers of chronic back pain.

fear avoidance
A form of behaviour that some people develop as a result of anticipation of pain on movement, coupled with the belief that such pain is harmful and likely to make the condition worse.

Processes that start out as quite natural, instinctive responses to pain can lead to a pattern of thoughts, beliefs and, therefore, behaviour that may lead to chronic back disability. Much research work in recent years has been looking at the factors that predict whether an acute back pain becomes chronic and disabling. Perhaps surprisingly, it is not the diagnosis or the severity of physical impairment that predicts whose back pain becomes chronic but is, in fact, issues such as negative thinking, catastrophizing and fear avoidance behaviour that are the strongest predictors of chronicity. Therefore, even if the latter issues apply only to a relatively small minority of acute back sufferers, early recognition and attention to this can make a big difference in the long run.

Be aware

During your moments of rest and modified activity, increase your awareness of your thought processes:

◇ Are you thinking along negative lines?
◇ Are you tense and bracing yourself against even small movements?
◇ Are you holding your breath when you start to move?
◇ Are you sweating and clenching your fists in anticipation of pain?

If you answered yes to any of the above you need to learn to relax the muscles, breathe slowly using your diaphragm in a gentle, even rhythm. Follow your train of thoughts and try to dispel the negative images, replacing them with positive ones. Even though you may not be entirely in control of the pain, at least you can be in control of your response to it.

Detached observation

Most people, when asked about their back pain, can say something about the movements and activities that either aggravate or relieve the pain. In fact, this information when elicited by the doctor or therapist often forms the basis of the practical advice they give the sufferer over the following days or weeks. For some, bending backwards may make the pain worse – for others, bending forwards or sideways is the problem. Prolonged sitting or driving often makes the back stiff, and the pain is worse on getting up out of the chair or getting out of the car, indicating that such activities should be limited or curtailed in the first few days after a severe back strain. Certainly, very few people are brave enough to engage in heavy lifting activities or digging the garden which involves a lot of back bending. At this stage of the process, to some extent the pain is a guide to modification of activity. For most people, following this guide, which can be worked out for the individual, leads to a normal process of recovery and relatively good return to function. It is only if you seek to completely avoid the pain by doing the minimum or next to nothing that you will face the risk of retarding your recovery.

During the first few days of an acute episode or recurrence of a familiar back pain, it is natural for your mind to turn to identifying the cause. Chapter 3 will go through the process of sorting out the likely causes. Very simply this can be divided into:

1 Simple or mechanical back pain.
2 Disc syndrome with nerve root involvement (pain radiating down the leg due to irritation or compression of one of the adjacent nerves).
3 Serious disease or **pathology**.

> **myth**
> Most back pain is due to muscular strain.

> **fact**
> Simple muscle strain or tear is actually a relatively rare cause of back pain.

> **pathology**
> Structural disease (as opposed to altered function which is reversible).

Q **My doctor says I have pulled a muscle in my back, but how could I have done that?**

A If the back pain came on after only a minor movement, it is unlikely, admittedly. Your doctor has probably identified an area where the muscle has tightened up, and is trying to reassure you that it is not too serious.

It is generally true to say that most back pain is caused by some problem with the joints of the spine. Muscles play a part either by splinting the painful level through increased tension (preventing movement of the painful joint) or simply becoming fatigued and aching in response to the abnormal posture imposed up on them. However, simple muscle strain or tear is, in fact, relatively rare when referring to the causes of back pain. It is of course quite common in the calf muscle or hamstring when playing sport. It is useful to gain some understanding of how the spine works in order to adopt a constructive strategy towards optimal use of the spine and body. Simply dismissing the back pain as a muscular strain along the same model of a pulled muscle in the calf is not particularly helpful.

myth
Severe incapacitating back pain must be a sign that something is seriously wrong.

fact
Less than 1 per cent of all back pain is due to disease or pathology – that is to say deep-seated infection, fracture of the bone, tumour, or crippling inflammatory disease. Any good doctor or therapist should be able to recognize the signs and symptoms and direct you to the relevant channels for further investigation. For the vast majority of back pain sufferers this is simply not necessary, and a quick reference to the self-diagnosis back pain flowchart in the Appendix should help to put your mind at rest.

In summary, one of the first roles of good back management is to understand the type of back problem you are dealing with in order to gain reassurance at an early stage.

Seeking professional help
(see also chapter 5)

The point at which a person should seek professional help will vary from one individual to another. The general guidelines are as follows:

✧ If, after following the initial advice for self-help in the first few days, your back pain is not improving, see your doctor or a registered physical therapist

◇ If the pain is severe and intolerable, and you cannot find any position for relief, you should naturally seek urgent help earlier, if only to gain some relief from pain

◇ If you are unable to control your bladder or bowels, feel numb in the saddle area or lose sexual function, see your doctor urgently

◇ If your problem has subsided to a manageable degree but keeps flaring up or continues to inhibit full return to normal activity, it is worth seeking professional advice either from your doctor or a registered therapist.

Q I have been going to the toilet to urinate more frequently – is that a cause for concern?

A Both pain and anxiety can cause this increased frequency, so don't worry as it is common.

If, by referring to the self-diagnosis chart in the Appendix, you seek professional help early, do bear in mind that it may be a false alarm.

Helping yourself

Here are a few useful suggestions for coping with an acute attack.

Relax

Find a comfortable position. Close your eyes and let all cares and worries evaporate. Deepen your breath and with each out breath let go of your muscle tension. It sometimes helps to let out a long audible sigh. To feel the rise and fall of your diaphragm, put your hands below your ribs and feel the expansion as you breathe in, and the contraction as you release the air. Start with your feet and gradually work up your body, letting go of any tension with the out breath. Finish with your throat, brow and eyes. Stay in this position for 20 minutes, observing the rise and fall of your breathing and the coming and going of your thoughts.

The Fowler position

If your back throbs in all upright positions, try 30 minutes rest in the Fowler position shown in Figure 2.3. If you find lying flat on your back uncomfortable, lie with your knees bent at right angles and your legs supported with pillows. This reduces the curve in your lower back and minimizes disc pressure. The lower back is relaxed and supported and the sciatic and femoral nerve roots are off the stretch.

Sleeping

For sleeping, try lying on your side with a pillow between your knees (see Figure 2.4). A small pillow between your knees prevents your hips from rotating and twisting your spine. A pillow at the head supports the neck at a right angle.

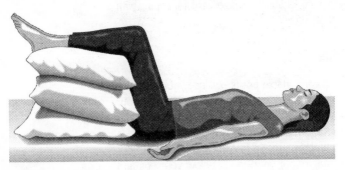

Figure 2.3 The Fowler position.

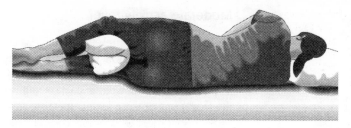

Figure 2.4 Lying on your side.

Massage

Ask your partner or a friend for a massage (see Figure 2.5). This is a simple 'stroking' massage of the muscles parallel to the spine. The thumbs apply steady upward and outward pressure in rhythmic movements up the spine.

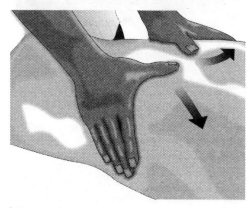

Figure 2.5 Massage.

Moderate activity relief

For short periods of relief between light to moderate activity, such as walking, try the knee hug position (see Figure 2.6). This position may help to relieve certain types of pain coming from the facet joints or tense lumbar muscles. Gently squeeze your knees towards your chest and relax. Repeat ten times.

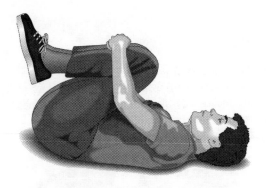

Figure 2.6 Knee hug position.

More active exercises

Once you feel like being a little more active, experiment with the following two exercises shown in Figure 2.7. Use whichever seems more helpful.

The Pelvic Tilt – breathe out and gently pull up with your pelvic floor muscles and in with your lower abdominal muscles. Press the small of your back flat. Hold for six seconds and repeat ten times.

The Passive Extension (McKenzie's) – slowly straighten your arms, relax your back and let your lower belly and pelvis remain in contact with the floor. Breathe in and out slowly. Lower yourself down and rest and repeat ten times.

(a) Pelvic tilt – starting position

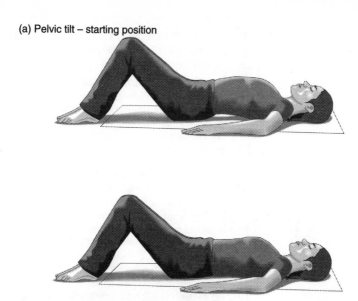

(b) Passive extension (McKenzie's) – starting position

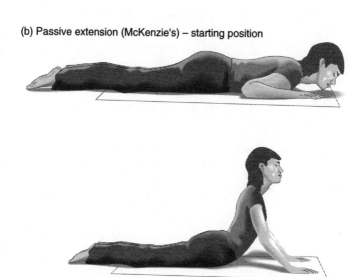

Figure 2.7 More active exercises.
a) Pelvic tilt b) Passive extension (McKenzie's).

A colleague of mine went to do a medical elective in Newfoundland as a general practitioner (GP). He recounted the following story:

After a few days of finding my feet, I was requested to make a home visit to a fisherman's cottage on the edge of town to see a man with severe gut pains. On being shown to the man's bedroom, I was shocked to see a pale, thin, pasty-faced middle-aged man lying in bed with curtains drawn. He had seen so little daylight that his skin had become almost translucent green. I asked him how long he had been in bed. The man replied 'Twenty years'. I asked what possibly could have prostrated the poor fellow for so long. He replied that 20 years ago he had visited his doctor in surgery with severe back pain from lifting some heavy fishing pots. He had been advised to 'go home and rest until the pain goes away'.

He said that the pain had been so bad initially that he had not dared to get up to test when or whether his back had improved. His wife had ministered to his every need, his fishing friends had helped them out, and this had gone on for 20 years. Not surprisingly he had become severely constipated – hence the gut pains.

If you've got back pain – don't take it lying down.

CHAPTER

3

Understanding your back and how it works

Diagnosing back pain

In this modern age of technology when we expect to have the answer for almost everything, it is natural to want to understand exactly what's wrong when your back is hurting. Advances in medical technology, particularly imaging, and expectations led by the media, encourage society to believe that there should always be an indentifiable cause for back pain.

However, even serious clinicians who research this question on a daily basis using painstaking clinical investigation methods cannot identify the source of pain in any more than 70 per cent of a population of patients with chronic low back pain. What's more, the knowledge and skills made available by these conscientious investigators have not yet been implemented by most doctors and specialists treating back pain for a variety of quite practical reasons such as availability of and access to resources, inadequate education or preconceived notions resisting change.

> **myth**
> Modern medicine should be able to find a specific, identifiable cause for back pain.

> **fact**
> Most back pain specialists admit freely that they do not know precisely what is wrong with 70–80 per cent of their patients.

X-rays

Traditionally, if a patient was not getting better, X-rays were ordered to rule out serious pathology such as bone cancer or infection, but also in the hope that the back pain could be ascribed to some visual abnormality seen on the radiographs. The most common 'abnormality' visible on X-rays is degenerative change. This means that a disc is narrow or the adjacent bones are showing signs of wear and tear by bone remodelling producing osteophytes. This is called 'spondylosis' derived from the Greek *spondylos* meaning 'vertebra' (see Chapter 1, page 7). In the past, many doctors and specialists, including complementary practitioners, would point to the area of wear and tear and say to the patient, 'this is the cause of your problem'. However, large-scale studies have shown that there is no correlation between the presence of degenerative disc disease (or spondylosis) and whether or not a person has pain. In fact, from the age of 18 or so, evidence of degeneration or age-related changes appear in the spine, particularly the lumbar spine and cervical spine. This increases with age such that by the age of 50, 50 per cent of the population shows these changes. In other words, they are so common as to be unhelpful in diagnosis. Since every X-ray requires exposure to ionizing radiation, and there are accumulative effects of radiation exposure throughout life, since the early 1990s there has been a strong move to reduce the unnecessary amount of X-ray investigation for common back or neck pain. In other words, the risk:benefit ratio for investigation of back pain with X-rays is simply not good enough to justify their continued use. Obviously there are some situations where X-rays are useful (see Chapter 6, page 97).

Magnetic Resonance Imaging

There are now non-ionizing imaging methods, such as Magnetic Resonance Imaging (MRI) and there is absolutely no harm to the body's tissues from lying in a strong magnetic field for half an hour. Furthermore, the images obtained give much more detail (see Chapter 6, page 99). However, once again, large-scale studies have shown that structural abnormalities, such as disc bulges and protrusions, appear commonly in the normal population (up to 35 per cent of people without back pain) as well as degenerative changes in their various forms. Quite often MRI scans do not improve understanding of the condition enough to change or improve the advice or treatment offered.

Moreover, at the present time MRIs are still relatively expensive and, in many parts of the world, a scarce resource. People are often disappointed when the MRI scan looks normal or simply shows normal signs of wear and tear for their age. Any changes that are found have to be related to the clinical picture, that is, the symptoms and physical signs obtained on examination, and then the MRI is useful. MRI is a more sensitive way of excluding serious pathology in the very small percentage in which such problems may be suspected.

myth
If my practitioner or therapist can't tell me specifically what's wrong, then I will need an MRI.

fact
This can sometimes be the case, but often an MRI will not be of any help and will only show what appears to be a normal scan for your age.

Precisely what is wrong with your back?

Returning to the fact that you want to know why your back is hurting, it is interesting to consider whether the exact cause actually matters.

An experienced doctor or therapist is able to rule out serious disease or pathology from examination, or from one or two tests if necessary. He or she can identify some of the more painful and debilitating causes of back pain

simple back pain
This refers to 'non-specific' back pain. The pain arises from a combination of different tissues in the body as well as mechanical factors which are too complex to fathom.

Q **If most common or garden backache is too difficult to understand why is it called 'simple'?**

A You may well ask. It is a medical sleight of hand. In truth it would be better termed 'complex' or 'multifactorial' back pain.

triage
A method first employed for military casualties in the Crimean war and now used to sort back pain into three useful categories requiring different approaches in management.

such as disc prolapse and nerve root entrapment purely from examination. The remainder can be grouped into one lump: that is, mechanical low back pain or common or garden backache, sometimes referred to as '**simple back pain**'.

When a patient visits a doctor with symptoms anywhere in the body, it is a common fact that 70 per cent of these symptoms come and go without accurate diagnosis or any real explanation. In other words, most general practitioners (GPs) are faced with this uncertainty on a daily basis. There is now a term for this called 'medically unexplained symptoms'. No one is denying the existence of these symptoms, i.e. the pain, its nature, its aggravating and relieving factors, but they are simply saying it is not possible in many cases to ascribe this to a specific cause, for example, injured tissue.

Does this matter? To the perfectionists among us, or those with a more obsessive trait, it may do, particularly if all efforts to help in terms of treatment for so-called mechanical/simple back pain are actually making little difference. Furthermore, it does matter to those people who are sufficiently disabled by their 'simple back pain' that they cannot lead a normal life. This book is not advocating ceasing the search for the causes of back pain, but simply advising you that searching for the cause may sometimes be fruitless, frustrating and often a distraction from getting on with the business of coping and trying to get better.

Triage

In the early 1990s, the advisory group on back pain, set up by the UK government, developed the concept of 'triage' when applied to back pain presented to the GP in primary care. Back pain triage divides people into three categories:

1 Those with suspected serious pathology (less than 1 per cent).
2 Severe nerve root pain (approximately 5 per cent).
3 Simple back pain (or neck pain) (approximately 94%).

In the less than 1 per cent category, clearly further investigation is required before any treatment or useful advice can be given. In the second category – nerve root pain – the priority is often to provide adequate pain relief since this can be very severe and demoralizing in the first few days or weeks. The most common cause of nerve root pain is disc prolapse in the middle aged. In the elderly, the most common cause is stenosis (see Chapter 4, page 74). The third group of simple back pain sufferers can be sub-divided by practitioners who are trained in manual palpation skills to enable them to apply specific forms of treatment. Additionally, with experience in treating back pain, there is a number of specific syndromes that experienced practitioners recognize (such as sacroiliac joint dysfunction). With the benefit of more than 20 years' experience in the diagnosis and treatment of back pain, I have developed the self-diagnosis flowchart (see Appendix). It is hoped that you will find your way through the self-diagnosis chart to obtain reassurance and guidance about whether to seek treatment, who to seek it from, and how urgently. Many of these syndromes are termed 'dysfunction'.

Q I have been given three different diagnoses by a chiropractor, physiotherapist and surgeon who all call themselves experts. Surely they can't all be right?

A No, there may be an element of truth in all of them, or probably two are wrong. Even 'experts' have their own perspective on back syndromes and, since there is little definitive proof available to disprove their theories on the diagnosis, you may continue to feel confused. That is why the term 'simple' backache can often feel rather reassuring.

What is a dysfunction?

The term 'dysfunction' is used widely in a number of different contexts. It refers to almost any system in the body, within human relationships or society, where there is a dynamic exchange of energy and force that is judged not to be functioning well or properly. It may be easier to use a sports medicine analogy to explain this. Athletes talk about developing their training programme to reach peak performance at the competition. The athlete and coach spend many months, often years, working out a programme of training and lifestyle balance that will lead to this peak performance so that on the day the athlete has the right mindset, fuel, co-ordination, power, speed, agility and whatever is required to produce their best. The same concept can be applied in other spheres such as performance in the theatre or playing a piece of music. Similarly, we can relate this to performing everyday tasks at work and at home in a way that is co-ordinated, efficient and minimizes stress and strain. In everyday activities we are not striving for peak performance, but hopefully for optimum performance. However, much of the time, for various reasons, we may not be performing optimally and we will constantly seek to adjust the various factors that we can control to reach this optimum daily performance.

We grow up and learn to take our bodily functions for granted, and only complain when things are not working properly. This could be due to neglect, misuse, disuse, overuse or actual breakdown of one of the component parts. In so-called 'simple back pain' or 'mechanical back pain', often a precise cause cannot be found, and structural changes can be ascribed to age-related change or degeneration equivalent to that of any other person of the same age. In this situation, the term 'dysfunction' is increasingly used, and it implies that the moving parts of the spine, or sometimes limb joints, are not functioning optimally. At some point when the function becomes too impaired, pain may arise even though there is no actual structural damage. For example, if you place your foot on a chair in front of you, leaving your knee unsupported and sit like that for more than 20 minutes, you are likely to experience aching and eventually quite severe pain in your knee. This is simply because you are placing the soft tissues around the joint under excessive gravitational strain. No actual damage has been caused and, as soon as you change position and gently move the knee, any stiffness will settle down, the pain will go and you can use the knee normally.

Stress and strain, muscle disuse or tension interact with our nervous system through reflexes in the spinal cord, the mind and emotions. This can lead to dysfunction of a spinal segment or region of the body, or sometimes our whole physiological system. This carries over to the rest of our life and leads to dysfunctional relationships with our partner, family and people at work. In turn, dysfunctional patterns or imbalances in these psychological and social areas of our life can affect the physiological workings of small areas of our spine or body on a 'micro' level. Some people find it hard to understand this concept, particularly if they are used to more concrete or black and white terms.

myth

If I take my car into the garage, the problem is simply a matter of finding the faulty part and replacing it so surely this should be the same with my back.

fact

This is not actually true if you look at this example in more detail. Any mechanic for a racing team can tell you that obtaining optimum performance from an engine is as much a matter of tuning and timing and getting the right fuel into the chamber at the right time as it is about actual breakdown or faulty components. It is helpful to understand how the spine works to see how dysfunction and these micro patterns of strain appear.

Q My osteopath says I have spinal somatic dysfunction. What does this mean?

A It is a term adopted by osteopaths after some important research from the 1940s. It indicates that the back problem is related to a complex of disturbances in the function of the nerves, muscles and joints of the spine, which are reversible. It does not imply damage or injury.

Structure and function of the spine

The spine has two main roles. One is to provide stability for the trunk in a variety of different postures, and the second is to provide protection for the central nervous system, i.e. the spinal cord. A third role is to provide a certain degree of mobility in order for our limbs to propel us with speed across the ground for survival reasons. As quadrupeds, the coil and recoil action of running on four limbs is a vital component to the speed and agility of fight and flight. As human bipeds, we still require a degree of flexibility for walking, running, throwing and other important but less dynamic everyday activities such as shopping, cooking, washing and playing golf. In some activities, such as domestic cleaning, there is a conflict between the balance of flexibility and stability that the spine has to maintain, in other activities like rowing (either bow or stroke position), the demands on the spine are too one-sided. In order to understand how things go wrong, it is important to know something about the normal structure and function of the spinal column.

Figure 3.1 shows a side view of the spine and a view from the back. From the side view, one can see a slightly 'S' shaped curve caused by the convexity of the thoracic area. Both the cervical spine and the lumbar spine have a natural concavity, also referred to as 'lordosis'. The lumbar vertebrae are heavier and thicker than the vertebrae higher up in order to support the greater weight. The spine rests on the sacrum, a triangular piece of bone which is wedged firmly between the iliac bones. Together these three bones make up the pelvis (see Figure 3.2). The thoracic area is somewhat stiffer, particularly on bending backwards and forwards, due to the

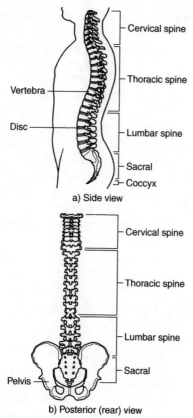

- Cervical spine
- Thoracic spine
- Vertebra
- Disc
- Lumbar spine
- Sacral
- Coccyx

a) Side view

- Cervical spine
- Thoracic spine
- Lumbar spine
- Sacral
- Pelvis

b) Posterior (rear) view

Figure 3.1 The spine.

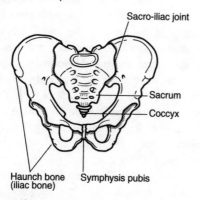

- Sacro-iliac joint
- Sacrum
- Coccyx
- Haunch bone (iliac bone)
- Symphysis pubis

Figure 3.2 The pelvis.

attachments of the ribs and the sternum which protect the vital organs. At the very top of the neck, there are two rather specialized vertebrae, the atlas and axis, which allow orientation of the head to facilitate vision and hearing. This area is also very important for balance and there are many fine postural muscles involved in the minute control of head and neck positions.

The spinal column consists of 34 segments, of which the last ten are mostly fused together, five in the sacrum which are fused and three to five parts in the coccyx which can have some mobility; these make up the tail bone.

Figure 3.3 shows a more detailed structure of a thoracic vertebra. The large, solid part is known as the 'body' which bears the weight vertically and helps resist compressive forces. The view from above shows the spinal canal through which the spinal cord and nerves run. A pair of segmental nerves emerges at each level to supply the muscle, joint structures and skin of a particular part of the body, leg or arm. In the early growth of the foetus, these segments are arranged very simply but, as the limb buds develop, these tissues push out into projections bringing with it their own segmental nerve. This results in a more complex pattern of **innervation** of the legs and arms. The vertebrae are joined together at the front by the intervertebral disc and at the back they interlock via the articular processes from above and below which together form the facet joint (or zygapophyseal joint). Small projections from the side of the vertebrae form transverse processes which provide sites of attachment for small and large muscles. Projecting from the neural arch – the ring of bone around the cord and nerves – are the spinous processes. These are the tips that can be felt and seen just under the surface, running down the centre of the back.

innervation
Nerve supply.

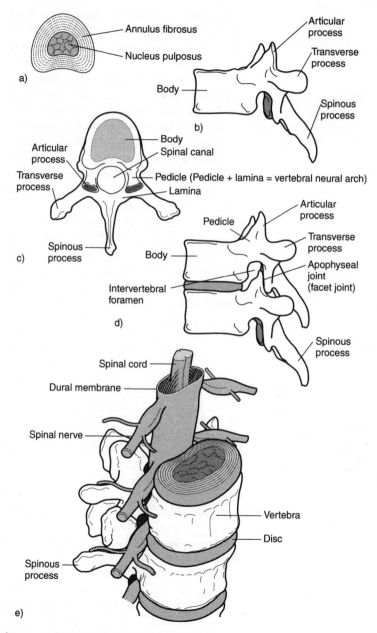

Figure 3.3 Thoracic vertebra.
a)–d) A thoracic vertebra e) A lumbar vertebra.

The disc has been the subject of much research in the last 50 years because it undergoes a process of degenerative change with age and also because it has been implicated as a significant source of back trouble since disc prolapse or **herniation** was first identified in 1934. The disc structure (see Figure 3.4), consisting of a tough outer fibrosus ring called the 'annulus fibrosus' and a gel-like centre called the 'nucleus pulposus', acts as a shock absorber, resisting compressive, shear and rotation forces due to the criss-cross pattern of fibre arrangement. This cushion allows a rocker like action of one vertebra on another. The disc derives its nutrition by diffusion through the specialized plates of cartilage lining the top and bottom of the vertebral body (endplates). So, the disc acts as a kind of joint but also as a cushion between each vertebra.

herniation
Another term for disc prolapse.

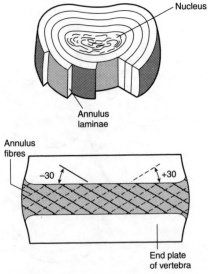

Figure 3.4 Intervertebral disc.

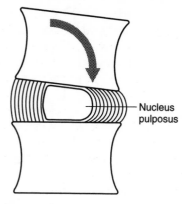

Nucleus
pulposus

Figure 3.5 The disc – a liquid ball-bearing.

The disc is extremely strong and is able to efficiently distribute forces by adapting its shape. It is sometimes described as a 'liquid ball-bearing' (see Figure 3.5). It mostly consists of water when young and gradually dehydrates with age. The outer fibrous layers contain some pain nerve endings. During upright weight-bearing activity, the disc is compressed, losing water and therefore height by as much a 10 per cent of its thickness over a day. The spinal discs need some recovery time to re-absorb fluid and nutrition. A night's rest is usually adequate. It is thought that, like other joints, the spine benefits from gentle and rhythmic activity, alternating periods of compression and rest in order to optimize its function.

The facet joints

The articular processes from above and below link together to form the facet joint (see Figure 3.6 on page 42). The facet joints have a layer of cartilage providing a smooth, friction-free surface, and a joint capsule containing a small amount of **synovial fluid**. By their arrangement, these joints tend to limit backward bending and

synovial fluid
Lubricating fluid that reduces friction in the joint.

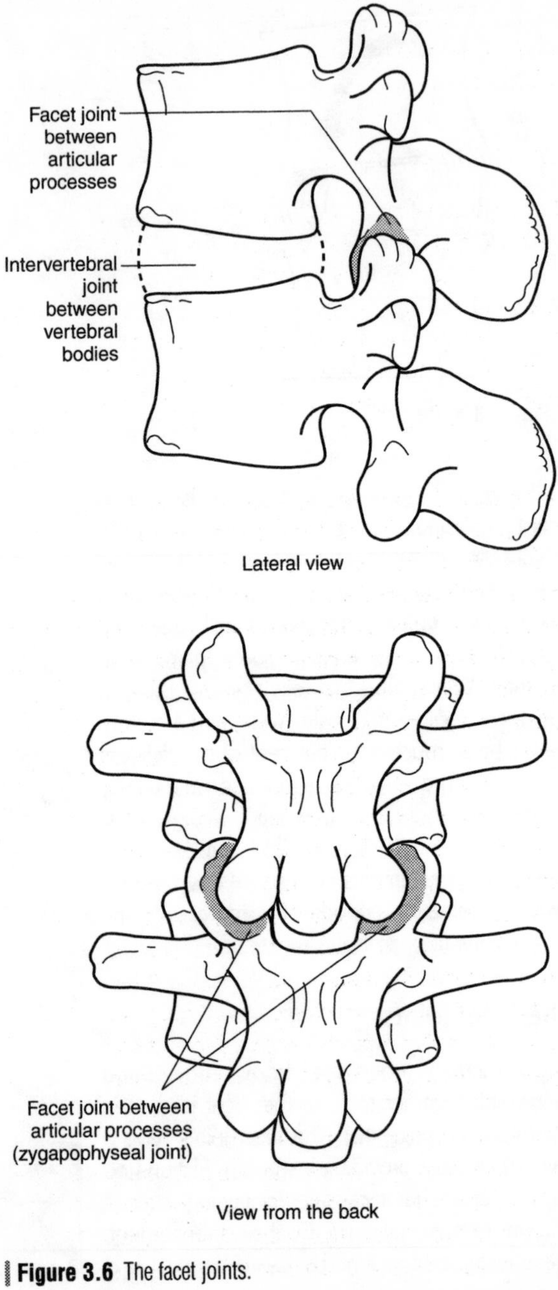

Facet joint between articular processes

Intervertebral joint between vertebral bodies

Lateral view

Facet joint between articular processes (zygapophyseal joint)

View from the back

Figure 3.6 The facet joints.

rotation movements. To some extent this protects the disc fibres which are not very good at resisting torsional strain.

The spinal canal

The spinal canal contains the spinal cord, which is a bundle of nerves passing from the brain to our extremities sending signals (Move! Hold! Relax! Adjust!) and bringing feedback from our senses (touch, heat, pressure, pain, stretch and position) to the centre of the brain. It is surrounded by membranes of which the outermost sheath is called the 'dura' or 'theca'. Within this dural sheath, the cerebrospinal fluid is contained, and this provides nourishment for the spinal cord and brain. The segmental spinal nerve (one of the pair of nerves that exits the spine at each vertebral level) is partly invested by this sheath as it leaves the spine through its own separate canal, which is called the 'intervertebral foramen'. Within this foramen, the nerve root widens (the dorsal root ganglion) because each nerve fibre has a cell body which is located at this site. The dorsal root ganglion is an important relay point for nerves coming from the disc, the vertebral body and its associated joints and structures, as well as the muscles, joints and other tissues of our limbs. At the lower end of the spine, around about the level of the second lumbar vertebra, the spinal cord ends and there is a fan tail of nerves which progress through to the sacrum and coccyx. This is called the 'cauda equina' because it looks like a horse's tail (see Figure 3.7).

The nerves need to be mobile within the canal, and in fact each nerve root can stretch several centimetres which is important to allow flexibility of our arms and legs. The lining of the nerve root, the dural sheath, is rich with nerve endings sensitive to pain and, when irritated by inflammatory chemicals, becomes even more sensitive to stretch or pressure. It is this membrane which is probably one of the main sources of pain in disc and nerve root problems.

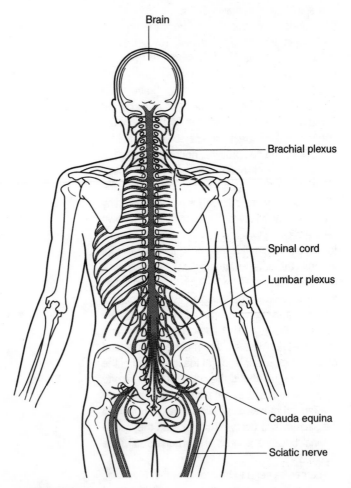

Brain

Brachial plexus

Spinal cord

Lumbar plexus

Cauda equina

Sciatic nerve

Figure 3.7 Back view of the spine.

The ligaments

The structure and architecture of the bones provide a hard restraint to movement, whereas the ligaments will provide a slightly elastic soft tissue restraint to movements.

In Figure 3.8 you can see a long, strong ligament in the front of the vertebrae (anterior longitudinal ligament), strong fibrous capsules around the facet joint, a long ligament running down the back of the vertebrae called the 'posterior longitudinal ligament', and further ligaments between the spinous processes, the intraspinous and supraspinous ligaments. These help to hold the bones together, providing a slightly elastic limit to the 'play' of the joint.

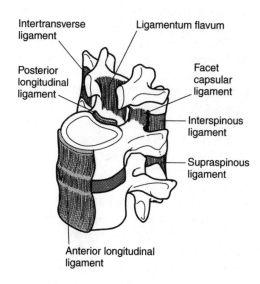

Figure 3.8 Ligaments.

In other words, they will allow certain additional or accessory movements such as gliding or sliding to a small degree. This gives the spine greater flexibility but ensures that the whole structure maintains integrity when put in extreme end of range positions. These ligaments are prone to sprain or strain and are richly supplied with nerve endings. They can be overstretched, in which case they lose their elasticity, or they can become thickened and scarred as happens to the yellow ligament (ligamentum flavum), possibly as a response to excessive play or movement when the disc is narrowed (due to degeneration).

The muscles of the back

Figure 3.9 shows the more superficial, larger muscles on the left side of the back and the smaller, postural muscles on the right side. The spine provides an anchor point for the large dynamic muscles such as the latissimus dorsi and gluteus maximus attached to the pelvis. The trapezius, which controls neck and shoulder movements, is attached from the base of the skull as far as the lower thoracic spine. These muscles are involved in moving the arm or leg. The spine needs to provide a stable base from which these muscles act. The smaller muscles include the multifidus at the back of the spine, the deep abdominal muscle layers – transversus abdominis – which wrap around the front, and even smaller muscles between each vertebra that act as stabilizers of the spinal segments. Collectively, the larger and longer muscles parallel to the spine are known as the 'erector spinae', literally translated as 'raisers of the spine'. It can be seen that the forces involved in holding a forward leaning position are extremely high since

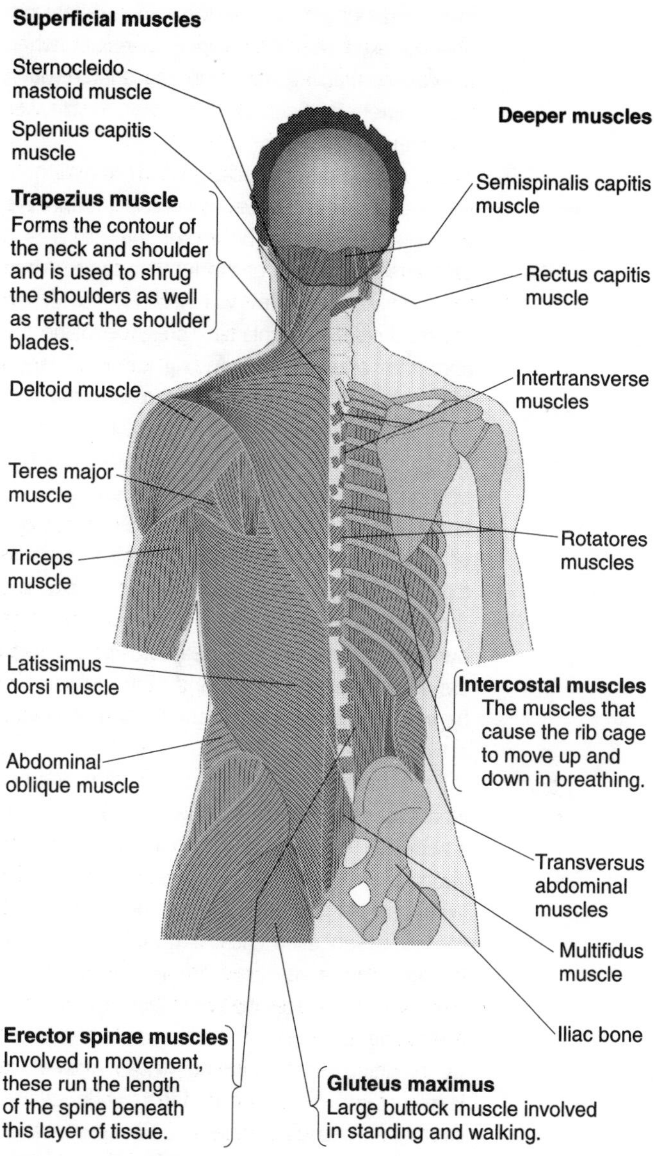

Superficial muscles

Sternocleido mastoid muscle

Splenius capitis muscle

Trapezius muscle
Forms the contour of the neck and shoulder and is used to shrug the shoulders as well as retract the shoulder blades.

Deltoid muscle

Teres major muscle

Triceps muscle

Latissimus dorsi muscle

Abdominal oblique muscle

Deeper muscles

Semispinalis capitis muscle

Rectus capitis muscle

Intertransverse muscles

Rotatores muscles

Intercostal muscles
The muscles that cause the rib cage to move up and down in breathing.

Transversus abdominal muscles

Multifidus muscle

Iliac bone

Erector spinae muscles
Involved in movement, these run the length of the spine beneath this layer of tissue.

Gluteus maximus
Large buttock muscle involved in standing and walking.

Figure 3.9 The muscles of the back.

these muscles act close to the spine and are not able to exert much leverage. Therefore, when they are contracting, the compressive force within the spine, particularly the disc, increases enormously.

The abdominal muscles, which form three layers, attach through various fascia (connective tissue sheet) to the bones of the pelvis and transverse processes of the lumbar spine. When they are working, they will help to provide an internal corset – maintaining pressure inside the abdomen and pelvis, providing counter-support to the spine from the front. When a person tries to lift a heavy weight, it is natural to take a deep breath. This will tense the intercostal muscles between the ribs, contract the diaphragm and tense the abdominal muscles. This is obvious when it comes to extreme weights, but much of the day we are doing small lifting and bending movements, unaware of the forces imposed on our spine. Some of these deep muscles, such as the transversus abdominis and multifidus, should be working almost continually in these everyday activities.

For a healthy back, all these muscles need to work together. For any muscle to work optimally, it needs to be able to relax fully, i.e. lengthen, and shorten up to one-third of its original length. When contracted, the blood supplied to the muscle is squeezed out. If a muscle stays tense for too long, it may start to hurt or develop a cramp-like feeling due to lack of oxygen. Sustaining a posture puts a muscle under strain, as in sitting with the head flexed forward, or leaning forward working under the bonnet of a car. When muscles are put under this sort of strain for a long time, they tend to become tight and weak, and fatigue rather easily. Therefore muscles, like joints and ligaments and discs, need regular movement and activity. In particular, they need to be stretched. Muscles are very sensitive to the chemical environment as well as the kind of nerve signals they are getting from the brain. It is now known that anxiety or fear can work directly on increasing the state of tension in the muscle. The connection between our mind and emotions and our body is instant and continuous. Since the muscles play such an important role in the overall health and function of our spine, we need to be aware of their needs in terms of relaxation and regular stretching.

Q The way the spine works is so complicated, why don't things go wrong more often?

A The beauty of our physiology is that there are instinctive and reflex patterns working beneath our conscious awareness all the time to maintain balance and harmony.

Muscle imbalance

It can now be seen that muscles work together to maintain posture and achieve movement. Both in the neck and shoulder region and the lumbar spine and pelvis, certain groups of muscles work together in patterns, and one can begin to identify the muscle imbalance pattern in somebody who sits a lot with their upper back rounded, their shoulders forward and their neck extended. Similarly, with regard to lower back posture, individuals who stand with their belly hanging out and increased lumbar lordosis (inward curvature), slack buttock muscles and pelvis tipped forward have an easily identifiable pattern of muscle imbalance. However, muscles are not simply important in maintaining static posture.

Spinal function

The term 'spinal column' gives the impression that the spine simply acts like a pillar of support for the rest of our body, and this can be misleading. Since we became *homo erectus*, our centre of gravity has shifted so that there is a vertical compressive force throughout the length of the body. The spine has had to modify and adapt (and has probably still got several million years of evolution to go in order to improve its adaptation to this new posture). Its structure is obviously essential to walking and to reaching and grasping objects. We not only walk with our legs, but in fact we use our whole back. When we talk and communicate, we tend to use our whole neck. When we touch, reach out, carry or throw objects, once again we are using our whole back. The pelvis has to transmit forces ascending each leg through its ring of bone containing one joint in the front, the symphysis pubis, and the two joints at the back, the sacroiliac joints. The shear forces through each sacroiliac joint as it bears weight on one leg and then the other in the normal **gait cycle**, are very high.

gait cycle
The pattern of movement of the legs when taking one complete step.

With running, the shear force is even higher. The ligaments across the sacroiliac joints and between the lumbar spine and the pelvis are the longest and strongest in the body. However, there needs to be a small amount of movement or 'play' for optimum function. It may well be that the ligaments in these joints help to store energy and return it in the cycle of walking and running. The lumbar region, consisting of five vertebrae, is mainly flexible in flexion and extension, enabling us to bend down and reach the ground. There is very little side-bending or rotation movement allowed in the lumbar spine, and a variable amount of backward bending. However, due to the arrangement of its facet joints, the thoracic spine is able to allow a reasonable range of rotation but, due to the ribcage, very little flexion (otherwise, expansion of the lungs would be prevented, restricting our breathing capacity). Nevertheless, even when you breathe, the ribs flare out and the spine slightly extends. When you breathe out, the thoracic spine flexes.

The bony structure of the neck is small but remarkably flexible. Since our head is relatively heavy, weighing between 6–9 kg (14–20 lbs), the muscles need to be relatively strong to support the weight whenever it deviates from a vertically aligned position. Within our **cranium** lie the sense organs to do with hearing, balance and vision. There is a complex system of feedback mechanisms between the nerves which control the small postural muscles in the neck and the information we are getting through our senses, so that small adjustments are continually being made. Most of the rotation in the neck occurs between the top two vertebrae, allowing 180° rotation.

cranium
The skull bones enclosing the brain.

my experience

I am a 37-year-old medical rep with three children, and I have been having back pain in my lower spine, mid-back and neck region, as well as some pain down one leg. I have to drive a lot in my job and then carry heavy bags of goods. I went via my doctor to an orthopaedic specialist who thought I might be having some disc trouble but it was not bad enough to require surgery. Eventually I found an osteopath who identified several levels in my spine at different regions that were not moving well. After a couple of sessions of manipulation together with some stretching exercises and advice on driving position I began to feel a lot better.

CHAPTER

4

How things go wrong

The flowcharts in the Appendix should give you an approximate idea of the possible cause of your back pain. However, it is difficult to be certain of some of these diagnoses with the usual investigations and even with specialist help. Many of them are arrived at through a combination of knowledge of spinal function, results of more recent research and clinical experience.

All too often, people are inclined to think that when something hurts, it means that something has gone wrong. However, prolonged muscle tension on its own can lead to a very uncomfortable, even painful, sensation and this is simply a result of prolonged static strain. Placing any of our sensitive soft tissues or even bones under prolonged strain can cause pain. Nothing has been damaged but the pain is simply a signal that excessive strain is being imposed on this particular region or muscle and it requires a change of posture.

myth
I have been diagnosed with back pain.

fact
Back pain is a symptom not a diagnosis.

Muscle tension

When muscles become chronically tense, they can cause **myofascial pain**. If an activity at work or at home involves constant repetition of the same fine movements of the arms and shoulders, for example, working on a production line, the muscles become fatigued. When this happens, the trigger points may form in designated areas in the muscles of your neck and shoulder area. Pain from these sites may then refer to other areas, either up into the head or down the arm (see Figure 4.1 on page 54).

Psychosocial factors may influence which individuals performing the same activities are most susceptible to developing headache, neck ache or shoulder pain. Anxiety, frustration and work overload may combine together to cause myofascial pain and dysfunction. Physical factors such as working with a cold down draught from an air conditioning unit – by cooling the skin and overlying muscles – can cause further tension, thereby reducing blood flow. Stimulants such as caffeine can increase the excitability of muscles, making them more liable to contraction. Disturbed sleep patterns and excessive alcohol intake, as well as hormonal abnormalities and some nutritional deficiencies can further increase the tendency for muscles to tire and tense more easily.

myofascial pain
Pain arising from the abnormal function of a muscle and its fascial covering. (The fascia is the sheath around a muscle which holds it together, keeping its shape and transmitting some of the forces.)

Trigger points

Not all **trigger points** are caused by repetitive strain or static postural strain. They may arise in an area of pain referred from a spinal joint where there has been mechanical dysfunction or derangement, in which case the spinal dysfunction requires treatment first. Obviously, it is important to alter any circumstances that may predispose you to trigger point formation, and this may mean checking your everyday routines such as your

trigger points
A 'knot' of hardened and contracted muscle that, when pressed or 'triggered' by various factors, refers to pain in a characteristic pattern.

workstation set-up. Think about your seating, the position of your monitor and keyboard, and the height of the work surfaces. These factors are collectively termed 'ergonomic', indicating the importance of the design of the workplace both in prevention and recovery from myofascial pain and dysfunction.

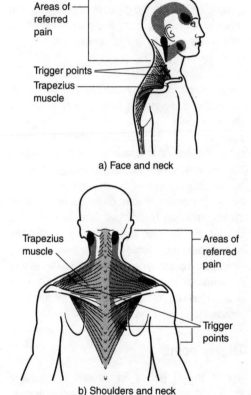

Areas of referred pain

Trigger points

Trapezius muscle

a) Face and neck

Trapezius muscle

Areas of referred pain

Trigger points

b) Shoulders and neck

| **Figure 4.1** Neck and shoulder area.

Muscle strain

Traditionally, many doctors have ascribed acute back pain to muscle injury because of the presence of muscle spasm. Most of the time the muscle reaction is secondary to the strain of the spinal segment, so this is not strictly accurate. Purely muscular injury is only likely to occur in a sportsperson undertaking vigorous exercise without sufficient warm-up and stretching. Extreme movements, which are uncontrolled or unco-ordinated, may cause some strain of muscles such as the large latissimus dorsi or some of the smaller erector spinae muscles such as the multifidus.

Muscle strain is obvious if there is bleeding and swelling, but most often there is simply strain of a few fibres resulting in a cramp-like sensation and localized spasm. Fortunately, these symptoms respond quite quickly to a combination of modified activity and exercise therapy.

Q What is good posture?

A Very few people are able to maintain an ideal posture, one which involves an efficient and symmetrical distribution of stress and strain throughout the joints and tissues. Any prolonged posture, even lying in the same position for too long, may put a degree of strain on muscles or ligaments. Hence the need for constant change of posture during a night's sleep. Patients with patterns of muscle imbalance, either affecting the neck or shoulder region or lower back and abdomen, can often be recognized by the way they stand or sit. Standing with the back hollowed for too long tends to overload the facet joints at the back of the spine. This may cause the classic 'cocktail party back' syndrome when you are constantly looking for a way to relax the back by perching on a stool, squatting or sitting down. Others stand with the abdomen and pelvis slouched forward in front of the centre line of gravity, causing a 'sway back' appearance. People with very lax ligaments and poor abdominal muscle tone are often prone to postural pain arising from the ligaments. Such a problem develops slowly and insidiously and may never result in acute episodes of pain but limits tolerance of standing or prolonged sitting.

fact
Discs do not, strictly speaking, slip, and neither do bones move out of alignment. The sensation that you are feeling, following an acute twinge of pain and a sensation of being stuck in a certain position with a cramping muscle pain or spasm, is due to a minor mechanical dysfunction in the spinal segment.

Spinal discs

Disc protrusion

Spinal discs can develop fissures through the annulus fibrosis (a specialized form of ligament consisting entirely of collagen) and may occasionally rupture and herniate (see below) in a dramatic way. This can produce severe pain in the back, and compression or irritation of one of the spinal segmental nerves. In these cases, pain may radiate down the leg in the lumbar region, or down an arm if this occurs in the neck. When a disc herniates, part of the nucleus protrudes through the crack or fissure in the annulus, breaking through the posterior longitudinal ligament into the spinal canal (see Figure 4.2).

disc protrusion
Protrusion of disc substance beyond the vertebral margins.

Disc protrusions are common and cause a variety of pains:

✧ Local pain and referred pain from an annular tear
✧ Referred pain from pressure on the posterior ligament or dural sheath
✧ Nerve root pain, or radicular pain, radiating down a limb.

The more severe protrusions or herniations tend to affect people between the ages of 30 and 55 because their discs have reached a stage of wear and tear when the annulus has become weakened and fissured. In the elderly, when the disc is more

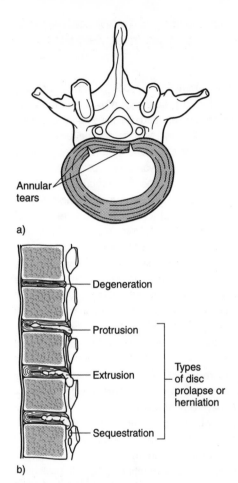

Annular tears

a)

Degeneration

Protrusion

Extrusion

Types of disc prolapse or herniation

Sequestration

b)

Figure 4.2 Disc abnormalities.
a) Annular tear b) Types of abnormalities

dehydrated and the pressure in the nucleus is lower, the disc is mainly fibrous so a large disc herniation becomes less likely, although it may still occur. Disc material from a **degenerating nucleus** is very inflammatory to the dura and nerve root, and tends to swell once it has escaped into the spinal canal, causing compression of the nerve. Sometimes this comes on without any real warning

degenerating nucleus

The pulpy centre of the disc (nucleus) undergoing denaturing of its proteins due to enzyme action.

because it is the result of the accumulation of stress and strain over many years, but at other times it may come on very acutely after an awkward bend or a heavy lift. In this situation, certain movements are painful and restricted – either forward bending, most commonly, or sometimes backward bending and sideward bending. You may find yourself deviated to one side or unable to straighten up fully, and the pain may increase when you sneeze or cough.

In some cases, the disc protrusion is severe enough that any degree of upright weight bearing is too painful, and a few days rest is required to take the pressure off. However, most of the time a certain amount of weight bearing is tolerated, and it now seems that gentle and regular activity may even encourage resolution of these problems. Very often prolonged sitting by virtue of the flexed position of the lumbar spine causes increased pain in the back or down the leg. **Radicular pain** or nerve root pain is called 'sciatica' when it occurs in the leg.

radicular pain
Pain due to compression or irritation of a nerve root.

It is important to remember that the pain is not necessarily down the back or side of the leg, but may sometimes radiate down the front of the leg when a disc protrusion has occurred at a higher lumbar level between the third and fourth vertebrae. In this position, sitting may appear to give relief whereas lying flat, whether supine or prone (face up or down), is extremely painful because of the increased stretch of the femoral nerve. Acute nerve root pain can be very severe, disturbing sleep, and it tends to affect about 5 per cent of all sufferers with back pain at some time in their lives. This is difficult to treat with simple physical measures, and may need pain relief treatments such as epidural injection and nerve root blocks for quicker recovery (see Chapter 6). Disc protrusions in the neck can occur gradually or suddenly, and tend to cause a similar pattern of restriction of neck movements. However, the radiating pain down the arm with sensory symptoms, such as tingling and numbness, usually indicate disc protrusion. In the thoracic region, disc protrusions do occur but tend to be less common and very rarely cause any nerve root compression. Occasionally, they can cause symptoms of cord compression, in which case urgent treatment such as decompression may be required.

Q My Uncle Jim slipped his disc at the age of 40 and never went back to work. Is this likely to happen to me?

A The natural history of disc protrusion or herniation is to recover with time. However, 10–20 per cent may continue to cause problems for considerably longer. Some of these may end up requiring surgery. However, the majority will resolve sufficiently to allow normal or modified activity but may be aggravated by heavy lifting, bending or any other situation that overloads the spine. In these cases, the piece of disc cartilage that has extruded has usually been absorbed but the pain continues to emanate from the internal disruption of the disc. This is called '**discogenic pain**' and results from sensitivity of the nerve endings in the outer layer of the annulus which continue to be aggravated by twisting or bending strains or simply by upright compressive forces. Inflammatory chemicals from the degenerating interior of the disc irritate the nerve endings and the whole structure behaves like a chronically strained ligament with delayed healing. People suffering in this way tend to fall into the category of chronic mechanical back pain and are unfortunately the ones most likely to become disabled. Active steps should be taken in the form of rehabilitation, and current research into newer treatments for discogenic pain will prove useful.

discogenic pain
Pain arising from within the disc due to internal disruption of the annular layers of fibres.

my experience

I developed an acute lower back pain at the age of 17 after lifting some heavy concrete blocks on a building site. My doctor arranged an X-ray which showed nothing abnormal. After a few weeks it did not go away so I went to an osteopath who spent some time mobilizing my back and taught me some exercises to do daily and the principles of good back care (how to lift and bend using my legs rather than my back). He said I probably had a small disc protrusion which would not show on a plain X-ray. My parents took me to see a specialist who arranged an MRI scan which did show a disc protrusion at the L5–S1 level (the lowest lumbar level between the bottom vertebra and the sacrum). He mentioned surgery was an option if it got much worse but I was getting better with the exercises. The worst pain on bending went away, but I continued to get back pain for many years on prolonged sitting and standing. I later went to a physiotherapist who found I had very tight back muscles 'in permanent spasm' and taught me pelvic tilt exercises and how to stand to reduce the tension.

This improved a lot over the next months and years but I still had back pain on prolonged sitting until I was able to afford a better car with good back support. Since then I have had periodic more acute pains on heavy lifting or violent twisting in sport, such as squash or tennis, but each time I was able to manage this with simple measures such as exercise and occasional manipulation. In my late thirties these attacks became more frequent and I wondered whether I should go back and see a surgeon. I was recommended to see a musculoskeletal physician who strongly advised at least a trial of prolotherapy injections to strengthen the supporting ligaments, before revisiting a surgeon. Fortunately this seemed to work very well and I have been relatively free of trouble for the last eight years although I still have to look after my back.

My conclusion is that the imaging investigations in my case made little difference to my management and, if anything, nearly encouraged the surgeon to do an unnecessary operation at one point.

Cauda equina syndrome

Although disc problems are painful, there is only one urgent situation – cauda equina syndrome. If you suffer a large disc extrusion in the lumbar region, on rare occasions it can compress the nerves controlling your bladder and/or bowels. If this happens, you will experience difficulty in emptying your bladder or loss of control of urine or faeces. You may feel numb in the genital or crotch area and this may cause sudden impotence. Any of these symptoms need to be brought to the attention of your doctor urgently because the earlier surgery is carried out, the greater the chance of nerve recovery.

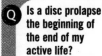 **Q** **Is a disc prolapse the beginning of the end of my active life?**

A Contrary to popular belief, disc protrusions and prolapses mostly resolve themselves in a few weeks or months, even without treatment. It is relatively rare that disc surgery is required.

Chronic nerve root pain

Although most disc prolapses resolve themselves, some people are left with a sensitive and irritable nerve that continues to play up in certain postures or on certain activities. This may occur even after disc surgery has been undertaken. Many people worry about the residual tingling and numbness in a patch of the leg, foot, arm or hand. Sometimes this continues long after the pain has resolved, and may indicate that a small part of the nerve has been permanently damaged. When a particular muscle or group of muscles supplied by that nerve has become weak, it usually recovers gradually over a period of six months to a year, but in some cases full recovery is not achieved. Most often this deficiency simply amounts to, for example, a slightly wasted calf muscle but can be more troubling if it leads to inability to raise the foot (dropped foot). Sensitized or damaged nerves can lead to the development of chronic pain syndromes with central sensitization (see Chapter 7, page 131).

Facet joint strain and dysfunction

Less severe episodes of back pain or neck pain may arise from an acute sprain of the facet joint with localized muscle spasm. This may occur because of an awkward or unco-ordinated movement or an acute compressive injury combined with extension and rotation. This kind of strain tends to cause back pain and possibly pain referred to the pelvic region, but very rarely is there much pain referred down the limb. It usually settles in a few days or, if prolonged, requires some competent manipulative therapy accompanied by exercises. In the older age group, a combination of wear and tear and similar strains may lead to a more chronic syndrome caused by all weight-bearing activity. This produces a constant, dull ache becoming more acute in certain postures when the facet joints are heavily loaded. It is usually relieved by lying down and does not conform to any particular pattern of movement restriction. This may be responsible for up to 40 per cent of chronic back pain in the elderly population and fortunately responds to a combination of postural retraining, facet joint injections and radio-frequency facet denervation (see Chapter 6, pages 107–9). Similar strains may occur in the thoracic region, affecting the joints where the ribs attach to the spine or the facet joints themselves. These strains are particularly well suited to manipulative therapy and rarely become a chronic problem. In the neck, these joints are larger in proportion to the whole spinal segment and more liable to be a cause of symptoms. In people who have suffered 'whiplash' strain involving hyperextension of the neck from a rear-end motor vehicle collision, these joints may be responsible for up to 50 per cent of chronic neck pain, and are amenable to the same treatment as facet joints in the lumbar spine.

> **Q** My therapist tells me that my sacroiliac joint is twisted or out of position. Since this seems to be a regular occurrence, will I have to keep going back for manipulation time and time again?

A The sacroiliac joint of the pelvis has been the subject of controversy in spine circles for many years. It is difficult to establish a precise diagnosis of sacroiliac joint pain without X-ray guided injection of the joint. In a fairly recent study of chronic back pain sufferers, it appeared to be the cause of pain in approximately 13 per cent of sufferers. Women with lax ligaments (sometimes called 'hypermobility' when it affects all the joints in the body) and women after childbirth are particularly prone to sacroiliac joint dysfunction due to relaxation of the ligaments. As explained in Chapter 3 (page 50), the sacroiliac ligaments need to be strong in order to resist the shearing forces imposed through walking and running since these are essentially one-legged activities (see Figure 4.3).

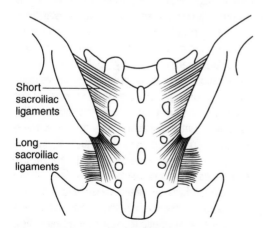

Short sacroiliac ligaments

Long sacroiliac ligaments

Figure 4.3 The short and long posterior ligaments.

The sacroiliac joint

The symptoms resulting from sacroiliac joint strain may be related to position or posture or may come on acutely with a sharp pain in the upper inner area of the buttock caused by a trivial jarring or jolting movement. The pain may be referred a little way down the leg or into the groin or side of the hip. Sometimes the strain may cause an apparent minor difference in leg length due to the very slight degree of rotation on one side of the pelvis and localized muscle spasm. Although the acute situation does respond well to manipulation, if the problem persists and recurs frequently, the ligaments will respond to stimulation by fibroproliferative therapy (see Chapter 6, page 109). An important but rarer cause of sacroiliac joint pain is inflammation in the joint as a result of some underlying systemic disorder. This can be related to gut problems, skin disease, infection elsewhere or ankylosing spondylitis (an inflammatory disease of the spine).

Unfortunately, there is no easy method of diagnosing 'sacroiliac joint dysfunction', which it is commonly termed, since imaging investigations do not help unless there is active inflammatory disease. Diagnosis is made from the history, physical examination by palpation, stress provocation tests and from local anaesthetic blocking of pain arising from the joint or ligaments. In young people, inflammation of the sacroiliac joint may cause morning stiffness and low back pain and may be the first sign of the inflammatory disease called 'ankylosing spondylitis'. This will only show on X-rays if the condition is fairly advanced, where the ilium and sacrum fuse together. It may show at earlier stages using magnetic resonance imaging (MRI), and special blood tests may assist in this

myth
The sacroiliac joint does not move significantly so is unlikely to cause pain.

fact
The sacroiliac joint has been shown to be capable of a small amount of movement, no more than a few millimetres, but certainly enough to be a source of pain. Some of the body's largest and strongest ligaments reinforce the position of the sacrum between the two iliac bones to withstand shearing and compressive forces. The sacroiliac joint is designed not to move too much and, although it has never been shown in any radiological studies to actually 'go out of position', there is no doubt that lax ligaments, as in people with hypermobility syndrome or during and after pregnancy, may cause significant pain and disability. In one study of patients with chronic low back pain, pain from the sacroiliac joint was shown to occur in 13 out of 100 cases.

diagnosis. There are a few other rare conditions in which the sacroiliac joint may become inflamed such as ulcerative colitis, Crohn's disease and Reiter's syndrome. There is also an association with psoriasis when joints are involved and other inflammatory disease of the spine commonly termed 'sero-negative **spondylo arthropathy**'.

In the more common mechanical syndrome of sacroiliac joint dysfunction, manipulation and stabilizing exercises provide the answer. Where the ligaments are insufficient to support the joint, the use of sclerosant injections, known as 'prolotherapy', may help. (Sclerosant refers to the solution more commonly used to harden and block varicose veins.)

spondylo arthropathy
Inflammatory joint disease of the spine.

Ligaments

The annulus fibrosis of the disc is a specialized form of ligament consisting entirely of collagen. Tears of the annulus, which may occur through cumulative wear and tear or by the whiplash mechanism from motor vehicle accidents, are known to occur quite commonly. In whiplash syndrome, the neck and head undergo violent acceleration/deceleration forces in which the weight of the head is first thrown backwards, compressing the structures at the back of the neck and stretching or tearing structures at the front of the cervical spine, and then forwards until the chin strikes the sternum, straining ligamentous structures between the spinous processes (see Figure 4.4 on page 66).

The articular surfaces of the facet joints and the ligamentous tissue of the capsules (the sac of fibrous tissue enclosing all joints and containing the lubricating fluid) have also been shown to be a significant source of pain in up to 50 per cent of chronic whiplash sufferers.

myth
Ligaments are not an important source of back problems.

fact
Ligaments can be a source of back problems, particularly associated with 'whiplash' and chronic sacroiliac joint dysfunction.

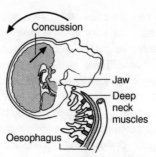

a) Head thrown backwards – shows structures likely to be strained

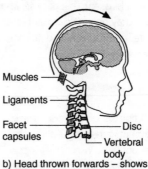

b) Head thrown forwards – shows structures likely to be strained

▌Figure 4.4 Whiplash syndrome.

Lower down in the spine, in the lumbar region where the disc narrows due to ageing and dehydration, the restraining effect of the associated ligaments is compromised, resulting in increased vertebral movement, one on the other. Although difficult to show convincingly (even with X-rays of the spine taken at the extreme of flexion and extension) because the amount of translation of one vertebra on another varies between individuals due to variations in ligament laxity, this does produce a clinical syndrome which has been referred to as 'lumbar instability'. Purists would argue that this can only occur when there is damage to bones or nerve structures. Most clinicians recognize the patient's account of constant background aching, worse with sustained postures such as sitting, frequent episodes of the back 'going out' or 'locking', resulting in a flare-up of pain with restricted movements. These commonly occur in the middle decades of life and make it difficult to engage in any prolonged bending or stooping activities. Straightening up from these postures often feels stiff and, in some way, blocked for the first few minutes. This type of back trouble is difficult since you will never feel entirely free of trouble. Attention to posture, general fitness and good muscle support is vital, and acute episodes can be treated by manipulation and mobilizing exercises. There is mixed evidence in support of the use of ligament sclerosants, known as prolotherapy, to strengthen the corset of ligamentous tissue around the vertebral segments. Occasionally, this syndrome becomes so severe that **spinal fusion** is considered.

spinal fusion
An operation to fuse two vertebrae together using bone or metal implants.

Spondylolisthesis

myth
When my back goes out, there must be a bone out of place.

fact
This myth is often perpetuated by talk of subluxations and putting vertebrae back into alignment. In the vast majority of these episodes, the symptom of 'something being out of place' can be ascribed to minor mechanical derangements or dysfunctions. This may involve movements of the nucleus of the disc within the different layers, moving through a tear or track into the outer, pain-sensitive part of the annulus fibrosis.

In a minority of back sufferers (less than 5 per cent), a lumbar vertebra is found on X-ray to have shifted slightly forward or occasionally backwards from its normal alignment. This is called 'spondylolisthesis' (see Plate 2).

There are basically two types of spondylolisthesis. The first takes place in childhood due to a bone defect in the neural arch called 'spondylolysis' (see Figure 4.8 on page 68 and Plate 3). If this occurs on both sides, then the normal arch of bone between the two articular processes no longer restrains the body weight from imposing a forward translatory force on the detached segment, causing a progressive forward shift of the vertebra. When children have this problem, it requires monitoring on a regular basis. Occasionally this shift progresses and requires fixation by surgical fusion.

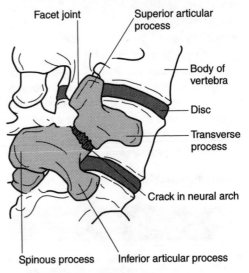

| Figure 4.5 Spondylolysis.

The second, more common, variety is the result of a wear and tear process called 'degenerative spondylolisthesis', affecting people over the age of 50, women more often than men, and African-Americans more than Caucasians. This results from a progressive elongation of the arch of bone between the two articular processes at the affected level, and progresses very slowly. This form of spondylolisthesis is unlikely to require surgical fusion unless there is nerve irritation caused by narrowing of the spinal canal. This progresses naturally to a stable situation in old age where the disc may narrow so much that there is effectively a natural fusion of the two vertebrae.

Childhood back pain

Back pain is relatively common in childhood and usually needs no further investigation. However, in the active young athlete who puts their back through repetitive compressive strain, for example, in fast bowling in cricket, there may be sufficient stress on the bony arch called the 'pars interarticularis' that a small fracture occurs – spondylolysis. This is often one-sided but may occur on both sides, usually at L4 or L5 (one of the two lowest lumbar vertebra).

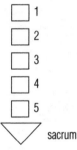

sacrum

Any reputable sports doctor will instantly recognize the need for diagnosis using appropriate imaging, usually high resolution MRI. The young athlete may require a period of rest from cricket or other sport they are playing too intensively, and they may need to engage in modified activities during a three- or six-month period of physiotherapy and rehabilitation. Surgical fusion is rarely required.

myth
Back pain in childhood is always serious and requires investigation.

fact
Backache is common in childhood and adolescence, affecting up to 15 per cent of the population in this age group, although usually only mild. In most instances it is the result of poor posture, disparities between skeletal and muscle growth, and common causes of strain and overstrain in the back.

I took my daughter, Desiree, who is a 15-year old junior gymnast, to see our GP about her back pain. She had trained in gymnastics two hours at a time, three days a week since she was nine. She had been doing very well until the last three months when she developed left-sided low back pain related to intensive tumbling practice on the mats. She had also had a fall off the vaulting horse which had shaken her a bit four months ago. She had been small, trimly built without an ounce of fat but had only recently started having periods and had grown 2 cm in height in the last six months. Her father and I were very proud of her talent and had great expectations for her future. The GP noticed that Desiree had a sharp lumbar lordosis, and winced with pain on extension, combined extension with rotation, and when standing on one leg leaning backwards. He also commented that she was very flexible. However, she was quite shy and never ate much despite her vigorous training. I did wonder where all her energy came from. Our GP thought it wise to check her back with an X-ray, and took some blood tests. The lab tests were normal but the X-rays showed a small bone defect at L5/S1 (spondylolysis) on the left. This seemed to fit with her clinical picture and he decided not to investigate further with a CT scan or MRI but recommended rehab with a physiotherapist who specialized in back rehab. He advised six months off the beam, vault and tumbling, but said that she could carry on with other aspects of gym training. This allowed the symptoms from the stress fracture at L5/S1 to settle. The physio found that her lumbar extensors were overactive, the deep abdominals were relatively underused, hip flexors rather short, and the hamstrings tight. He concentrated on improving her muscle activation in weekly sessions to build up her core stability. He gave her a home exercise programme, which she did conscientiously. During the six months relative lay-off, Desiree had time to develop other interests. I was very pleased that her appetite improved and she seemed to enjoy life more. She returned to gymnastics but eventually decided to pursue a new interest in jazz dancing.

osteochondritis
A disorder of the edge of the vertebra (growth plate) or ring of bone in adolescence, causing irregularity and alteration of vertebral shape.

Another important cause of back pain in childhood is called 'Scheuermann's Disease', a form of **osteochondritis** (see Plate 4) affecting the growth plates of the vertebrae. This occurs during adolescence and is easily identified on X-rays by the irregular, slightly moth-eaten appearance of the vertebral endplates (see page 40) and the wedged appearance of the front of the vertebrae in the thoracic region.

This process may occur silently without producing symptoms, but in the active athlete may cause diffuse thoracic/lumbar pain, aggravated by excessive activity. If the youngster is allowed to continue their activities, usually swimming or gymnastics, then a progressive kyphosis or **flexion curvature** of the thoracic spine may develop. This is best treated by avoidance of the aggravating activities and corrective postural exercises. This rarely develops to a point where surgery or spinal bracing is required.

flexion curvature (kyphosis)
Increased convexity of the spine (it is naturally slightly convex – backwards.

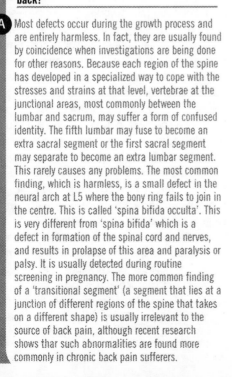

Q The X-rays taken of my spine show a bony abnormality – does this mean I have a weak back?

A Most defects occur during the growth process and are entirely harmless. In fact, they are usually found by coincidence when investigations are being done for other reasons. Because each region of the spine has developed in a specialized way to cope with the stresses and strains at that level, vertebrae at the junctional areas, most commonly between the lumbar and sacrum, may suffer a form of confused identity. The fifth lumbar may fuse to become an extra sacral segment or the first sacral segment may separate to become an extra lumbar segment. This rarely causes any problems. The most common finding, which is harmless, is a small defect in the neural arch at L5 where the bony ring fails to join in the centre. This is called 'spina bifida occulta'. This is very different from 'spina bifida' which is a defect in formation of the spinal cord and nerves, and results in prolapse of this area and paralysis or palsy. It is usually detected during routine screening in pregnancy. The more common finding of a 'transitional segment' (a segment that lies at a junction of different regions of the spine that takes on a different shape) is usually irrelevant to the source of back pain, although recent research shows thar such abnormalities are found more commonly in chronic back pain sufferers.

Curvature of the spine

Q My therapist says I have an abnormal curvature in the spine. Is this something to worry about?

A No, in most instances, you do not need to worry. Rarely, it will need to be monitored, except in children where it might develop further.

A therapist may detect a small variation from normal spine curvature, manifested by a slight lateral bend in the spine in the thoracic region or thoracolumbar region (junction of thoracic and lumbar region). Occasionally, such a curvature may be isolated to the lumbar spine alone. A gentle 'C' shaped curvature throughout the whole length of the spine is usually a result of the pelvis being tilted to one side due to a difference in the length of your legs. This is probably the most common cause of curvature since up to 10 per cent of the population have up to 1 cm (0.39 in) of difference in leg length. The therapist is trained to identify these small differences in symmetry of the spine. However, these minor variations from perfect symmetry usually bear little relation to the cause of back pain. But if you have a young child or adolescent who has a significant hump or obvious asymmetry in their trunk, this will become more marked when they bend forward, and show as a rib hump. This is a true structural scoliosis which can progress during growth to become quite severe. This should be followed on a regular basis by a specialist in scoliosis who will usually recommend postural exercises and occasionally spinal bracing, although it has not been established if this makes much difference to whether the curvature progresses. If the curvature progresses to more than a 45° angle, surgery may have to be undertaken.

Most people have minor curvatures which do not require routine monitoring. However, more moderate degrees of curvature may progress insidiously in later life and lead to postural pain and problems. Very occasionally, these may require correction in adulthood. The isolated lumbar curvature usually causes no problem until you are old when progressive wear and tear of discs leads to unequal pressure on the facet joints or narrowing of the nerve root canal. This situation can lead to chronic back pain.

Back pain in older people

Despite the fact that more people tend to get back pain during their middle years compared to when they are older, there is recent evidence from studies that with our ageing population, back pain is still relatively common. Facet joint disease due to wear and tear certainly rises to an incidence of up to 40 per cent of the total back pain population in over 65-year olds. This is recognizable from the typical history of pain from upright activity which is relieved by rest and not particularly provoked by any specific movements as it is with disc problems.

However, with ageing and wear and tear comes narrowing of the disc. As the vertebrae settle one upon the other, the spinal canal may narrow both centrally and in the nerve root canal laterally (see Figure 4.6 on page 75). This figure also shows a spinal canal that is narrow from birth (congenital). This predisposes individuals with congenitally narrow canals to problems earlier in life. If a disc herniation or protrusion is also present the canal is further narrowed. Development of **osteophytes** from facet joints and the vertebrae may also encroach on the canal space, see Figure 4.7 on page 76. Instability may lead to thickening and scarring of the yellow ligament, further narrowing the central canal space. This leads to the syndrome of 'spinal stenosis', when the canal is so narrowed that the blood supply to the nerves is constricted. This commonly occurs at one or more levels in the lumbar spine. In practical terms, this will mean that a person will prefer to walk stooped or pushing a shopping trolley or child buggy rather than stand and walk upright. Their walking distance

Q My doctor says my back pain will improve when I get older – is this true?

A Because the disc is beginning to wear, people get more trouble during their middle-aged years due to the natural history of disc degeneration and periodic protrusions and prolapses. In the elderly, the discs have become stiffer and dehydrated and are much less likely to prolapse.

osteophytes
Outgrowths of bone resulting from remodelling and adaptation to stress and ageing.

will become progressively shorter due to the development of back pain and leg pains, sometimes accompanied by a feeling of abnormal sensations in the legs. People often say 'my legs don't belong to me' or 'they feel heavy and weak'. This feeling of lack of balance and control will cause the person to sit down or bend over and stoop. This seems to produce almost immediate relief. People often say they can cycle for 8 km (5 miles) but can only walk for 200 m (650 yards) before the symptoms come on. This is because when you are sitting, the lumbar spine is flexed, widening the canal. This allows enough room for the circulation to reach the nerves. In our ageing population, this condition is becoming more and more common. It is important to distinguish this from the other common condition affecting walking distance in the elderly, that of poor circulation in the legs causing 'claudication', which is the cramping of the calf muscles. Vascular claudication refers to circulatory impairment due to a narrowing of the blood vessels in the pelvis or legs. This narrowing of the blood vessels is caused by clogging or furring of the arteries with fatty deposits. Neurogenic claudication refers to reduced blood flow to the nerves in the lumbar spinal canal due to narrowing of the spinal canal.

Lateral canal stenosis

Sometimes the narrowing occurs only in the root canal (**intervertebral foramen**) due to bony overgrowth as a result of wear and tear. This may produce pain in the distribution of one nerve root in the leg, but is similar to central canal stenosis brought on by upright activity, standing and walking. Both these problems tend to progress slowly with age and simple adjustments are using a stick and accepting the need to stoop in old age.

intervertebral foramen
The lateral canal through which the spinal nerve root emerges.

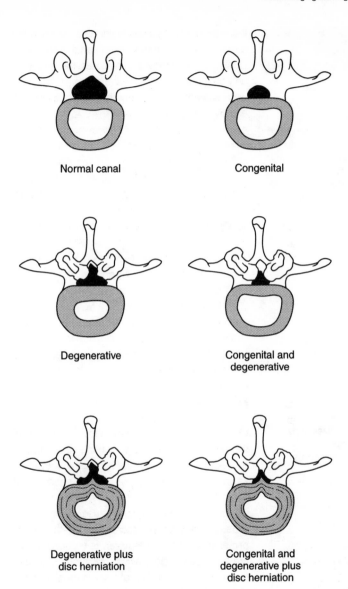

Normal canal

Congenital

Degenerative

Congenital and
degenerative

Degenerative plus
disc herniation

Congenital and
degenerative plus
disc herniation

Figure 4.6 Canal space.

fact
Although it is the most common affliction of the elderly spine, osteoporosis is not universal. Osteoporosis receives much attention in the media, and research in recent years has been done into the causes and treatment of this debilitating condition.

If it is more severe, steroid injections placed in the spinal canal or nerve root canal may help. However, in the most severe cases, this help may only be temporary and decompression of the canal with surgery is the only means of obtaining effective and long-lasting relief.

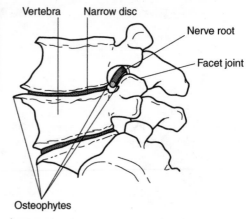

Vertebra   Narrow disc

Nerve root

Facet joint

Osteophytes

Figure 4.7 Osteophytes – constricting the lateral canal or nerve root foramen.

Osteoporosis

Q My back hurts, could it be osteoporosis?

A Many people mistakenly believe that osteoporosis in itself is a cause of pain. In fact, bone demineralization tends to occur to a greater or lesser extent with age and declining activity. It is not painful unless there is an actual fracture or collapse of the vertebra.

Osteoporosis is the progressive loss of strength of the bones due to the rate of bone re-absorption exceeding the rate of bone rebuilding. Inevitably, as we get older, we lose height, but rapid loss of height with increasing kyphosis may be a sign of osteoporosis. After the menopause women are at increased risk of osteoporosis since the bone-preserving effect of oestrogen is reduced. There are hereditary factors which make some people more liable to rapid loss of bone mineral content and smoking, being fair-haired and slight of figure, inactivity, and oral steroid use for other conditions will increase the risk of osteoporosis. Some women never achieve a reasonable peak bone mass, even in their twenties, due to menstrual abnormalities, anorexia, poor diet, lack of regular exercise or excessive exercise.

Men are more fortunate in that the only significant risk factor is the normal process of ageing and declining testosterone production. However, malabsorption may affect either sex due to chronic digestive diseases, and it is advisable that all people at risk supplement their regular diet with calcium and vitamin D. Hormone replacement therapy (HRT) may help if there are no risks attached.

Anyone at significant risk should ask their doctor for a baseline bone density measurement so that monitoring can be maintained. In people at risk, the use of special bone mineralization hormones, such as bisphosphonates, can be started early to reduce the risk of spine or hip fracture. There are one or two metabolic diseases of bones which may lead to weakness and vulnerability to compression. These include Paget's disease (a metabolic disturbance affecting the structure causing enlargement at the expense of strength) and osteomalacia (a result of inadequate vitamin D absorption). Vitamin D is partly manufactured in the skin as the result of exposure to sunlight, and it is now recommended that everyone should obtain at least half an hour of exposure to sunlight every day, weather permitting.

Compression fracture is perhaps the most commonly missed diagnosis in the elderly because many doctors and therapists still do not recognize the characteristic history of an acute osteoporotic collapse of the vertebrae (see Figure 4.8 and Plate 5). Usually the pain is severe and radiates right round in a girdle-like fashion. If it occurs in the thoracic region, then it is certainly difficult to breathe. Movement in any direction away from neutral hurts. Sitting down, getting up and turning over in bed is agony. There is much associated muscle spasm and extreme tenderness on direct

Q I stooped to pick a pin off the floor and have had severe back pain ever since, making it difficult even to breathe. What should I do?

A If you are over 65 and can identify any of the risk factors for osteoporosis, it is possible that the insidious process of demineralization of your spine has weakened the structure so much that even a bending and lifting activity can cause vertebral collapse.

palpation or percussion at the affected level. X-rays will usually identify the problem but it may not be very clear when there has only been a partial collapse. Sometimes a bone scan or CT (computerized tomography) scan is more useful.

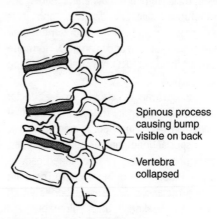

Spinous process causing bump visible on back

Vertebra collapsed

Figure 4.8 Vertebral collapse.

Q I'm still not sure of the cause of my back pain.

A You can use the flowchart in the Appendix to arrive at a common syndrome or possible cause or condition. This may also point to certain specific actions or reassure you that there is no immediate cause for concern or action. If, however, your pain experience does not fit any of the common syndromes, certain features may alert you or your doctor to seek investigation. Severe, unrelenting pain in people under the age of 20 or over the age of 60, which is occurring for the first time in your back, and is not settling in a few days or weeks, needs investigation. This is especially important in the following situations:

✧ If the pain is not affected by any movement or posture, and is constant and gets worse at night when you are resting; this may be a sign of non-mechanical pain due to other causes
✧ If you have a past history of cancer

A
- ✧ If you are feeling generally unwell and losing weight with an unexplained loss of appetite; this can indicate more serious disease
- ✧ If you have developed an obvious swelling or deformity in your back; this requires investigation
- ✧ If there is widespread weakness or numbness in your legs or arms, see your doctor
- ✧ If you have been unwell with a systemic infection or are known to be HIV positive or perhaps already suffer from AIDS then your back pain may not be as simple as you would like to think
- ✧ Pain in the thorax is common and usually benign, but because within your thorax there are so many organs which may refer pain to the back, your doctor will investigate this further.

my experience

I am a 44-year-old printer and I had been having some pain radiating down my left leg on and off for a few weeks. I awoke one morning with severe back pain and increased pain in my left leg. After a day in bed I tried to get to see my doctor but could not get into my car because it hurt to bend even my head. So I called the doctor out to see me. I told the doctor I had been lifting some heavy printing equipment a few days earlier and had felt a twinge in the centre of my lower back but thought nothing of it. The doctor said I had severe limitation of movements and prescribed me painkillers and exercises. Over the next 24 hours the pain got worse so that I could no longer walk to the bathroom. I now had pain down both legs and called my doctor again when I found I could not pass urine. The doctor sent me to the hospital accident and emergency where I was admitted and an MRI scan was ordered. This showed a large central disc prolapse at the fourth lumbar level. Surgery was arranged urgently to remove the disc fragments from the spinal canal as they were compressing my nerves to the legs and bladder.

After surgery I was able to pass urine normally, although my legs were a bit weak. However, I had some physiotherapy and over the next few weeks my full strength returned.

CHAPTER

5

Who should I see?

In Chapter 2 we covered the initial steps of self-help with acute back pain. This may be sufficient for most patients and, if fortunate, the problem will clear very quickly and everyday activities and work can recommence. However, if you have had a second or third episode which is not clearing up as fast as previously, or there is a concern about the recurrent nature of the problem, then you should consider consulting a specialist for further help. If this is the first episode and all the self-help measures are not improving the situation, it is natural to look for further help. If the pain is so severe, for example nerve root pain or sciatica in the leg that cannot be controlled, then it is perfectly reasonable to want to seek expert help.

In the UK, a general practitioner (GP) – the family doctor – is the first port of call for most non-emergency conditions. The vast majority of people are signed on with a GP in their neighbourhood and should have ready access to his or her knowledge and skills.

The doctor's approach

All GPs in the UK have been educated to fulfil essential tasks when dealing with back pain. The triage approach sorts the problem into one of three categories:

1 Pain requiring further investigation [looking for 'the **red flags**' that may indicate more serious disease and picking up any '**yellow flags**' (psychosocial factors) that indicate a risk for the problem becoming chronic]
2 Nerve root pain
3 Simple back pain.

In order to use the triage approach, the doctor will take a history of the complaint. This involves taking down details of the pain, its duration, distribution, aggravating and relieving factors, nature of onset and severity. He or she will also take into account any previous medical history which will be on record. He or she will then examine you, and for this you will need to undress to your underwear. You will be assessed, initially standing, in order to record the range of active movements in backward bending, bending sideways in each direction and forward bending. The doctor will ask where the pain is located and which movements hurt and, if so, where. He or she will note down any restriction of range of motion. If there are referred pains or nerve root symptoms in the limb, the doctor will also examine the reflexes, sensation and muscle strength, and whether the pain is in the arm or leg. For the lower back assessment, the doctor will assess you while you are lying down, in particular performing the straight leg-raising test, and looking for signs of restriction and nerve root tension. He or she should also examine your hip joints for restriction of movement. Lying prone, the doctor will gently palpate and spring the

red flags
These are the symptoms such as unexplained weight loss that may indicate more serious underlying disease and would prompt your doctor to investigate or refer.

yellow flags
The term coined for the psychosocial factors (stress, depression, negative beliefs and fear of moving) that are risk factors for becoming chronically disabled.

Q My doctor tells me not to rest but it is so painful doing anything else I really haven't got any choice.

A He is following the guidelines on management. Many studies, although not all, have shown that rest does not help recovery in the long run. In the short term (for a few days), unloading the spine eases the pain and reduces muscle tension and, rather than being harmful, may actually help.

lumbar segments and sacroiliac joints, assessing for local tenderness and muscle spasm.

If your doctor is concerned about there being more serious disease, he or she may arrange for some blood tests or for referral for a second opinion. However, in the vast majority of cases, this is unlikely to be an issue since less than 1 per cent of people with back pain have any serious underlying pathology. At this stage, the doctor will be able to decide what category or group of back pain sufferers you belong to and advise on the appropriate action. If there is a physiotherapist available, or if there is easy access to local physiotherapy, the doctor may recommend a visit to initiate some active treatment. Before doing this, he or she will of course spend some time explaining the nature of the problem and how to best look after your back in the immediate future. He or she will hopefully be able to provide reassurance about the benign nature of the problem and the expected natural recovery. He or she will probably advise against any prolonged bed rest since it has been shown to do more harm than good. Instead he or she will advise sensible modification of activities such as reduced lifting of heavy weights and manual work until you have improved.

Your doctor may have a simple exercise sheet for you to initiate some gentle mobilizing and strengthening exercises. He or she will probably be able to quote commonly used statistics on the recovery rate from acute, simple back pain if this is the group that you fall into. The statistics are that 50 per cent of patients improve within two weeks and 90 per cent within four to six weeks (although complete recovery may take longer). He or she should advise you to return to work as soon as you possibly can, even if that means on light duties or a modified work routine in the first instance. He or she may be willing to certify you as unable to work for a few days, or a week or two at the most.

In addition, your doctor may prescribe simple painkillers such as paracetamol, anti-inflammatories (ibuprofen) and/or muscle relaxants (diazepam) for short-term use. All of these have been shown to be useful in aiding recovery.

Your doctor may also give you a little booklet called the *Back Book* which serves to underline these important messages.

Currently most patients will rarely see their doctor more than once for a back pain episode, but ideally the doctor should review a patient's progress at about 10–14 days from the onset to check that they are making good progress. If not, the doctor will recommend an appointment with a physical therapist (see below).

myth
Ninety per cent of acute back pain episodes are alright after six weeks.

fact
Recent follow-up has shown that this is simply not true. Even 12 months later up to two-thirds of patients may have some pain and disability.

my experience

As a 33-year-old mum of two, I visited my GP with acute low back pain of seven days which restricted my ability to bend, lift and pick up my children. I was working part-time as a nurse and my husband was away a lot on business. I had no other help at home and was feeling anxious about my ability to cope, and I had also been low in spirits since the birth of my last child eight months ago. This pain had been severe initially and I almost got stuck on the toilet in the middle of the night, unable to get to my baby who had been crying. My GP, having listened to my account, examined me and found evidence of 'simple mechanical back strain' with no nerve root involvement or 'red flag' signs. He noticed that I was very anxious, I was holding my breath on movement, afraid of the pain, and hypersensitive in certain areas of my back and buttocks on deep palpation. He explained that I had been overdoing it and strained my back. There was nothing seriously wrong. I asked whether an X-ray could be done since I was concerned about the reliability of my back. He explained that this would not help either with diagnosis or finding the best way to manage my problem. He gave me a home exercise sheet and arranged for me to see the practice physiotherapist as soon as possible. I started to move around the house more confidently, taking care to kept my back straight while lifting my baby. By the time I saw the physiotherapist a week later, I had less pain and less anxiety but still felt generally low and worried about the future. The physiotherapist examined me and gave the same reassuring messages as the GP. She then massaged the tender soft tissues, and listened to me talking about my rather stressful and lonely life. She empathized strongly, having had some similar life experience and described how the first five years of motherhood had been so difficult but now that she was through it, it all seemed worthwhile. The physiotherapist said that what helped was that she decided that however busy she was, she would insist on doing something she enjoyed just for her, for half an hour each day. This might be exercises to a home video, relaxing to music, going to see her sister for a chat or just getting out for a good walk with the buggy. The physio mobilized my lower lumbar levels directly and taught me some specific McKenzie exercises – passive extensions to do frequently and regularly. A week later I returned to the physiotherapist feeling much better and told her that I had had a good talk with my husband, expressing how I needed him to be around at home more. He was going to talk to his boss about reducing his travel commitments and I felt so much happier.

Severe nerve root pain

If your doctor finds evidence of nerve root irritation accompanied by severe pain, or evidence of nerve root compression with loss of tendon reflex, weakness in certain muscles and loss of sensation, he or she will certainly prescribe you some strong painkillers. These could include codeine-based medication or tramadol plus non-steroidal anti-inflammatories if you do not have any history of indigestion or peptic ulceration. Your doctor may be able to arrange a fast track referral to the acute pain service for epidural or nerve root block with corticosteroid (steroids such as cortisone). If such a service is not available, or there is a long waiting list, there may be a local doctor with a special interest in musculoskeletal conditions, an orthopaedic or musculoskeletal physician, who will

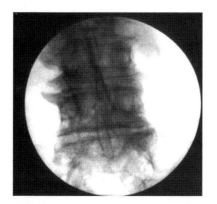

Plate 1   Spondylosis

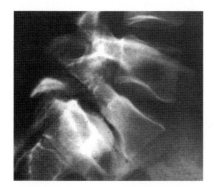

Plate 2   Spondylolisthesis.

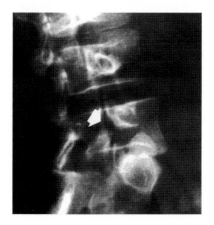

Plate 3   Spondylolysis.

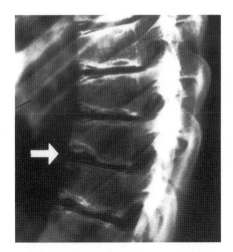

Plate 4 Osteochondritis.

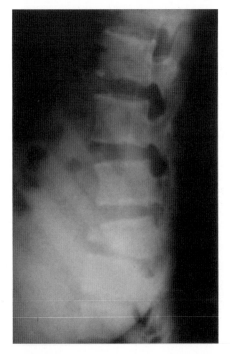

Plate 5 Vertebral compression fracture.

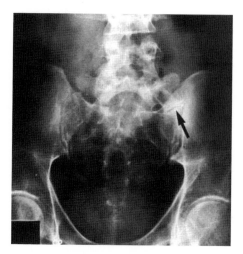

Plate 6 Bony anomaly.

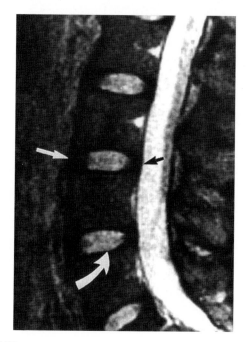

Plate 7 Normal MRI scan.

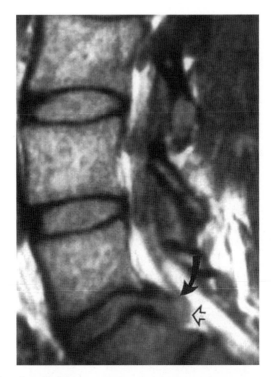

Plate 8 Disc prolapse side view.

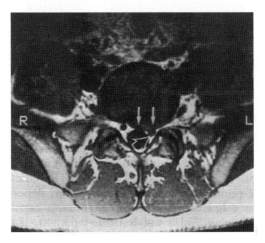

Plate 9 Disc prolapse cross-sectional view.

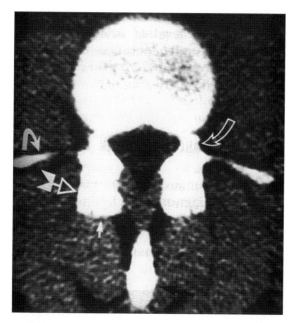

Plate 10   Normal CT scan.

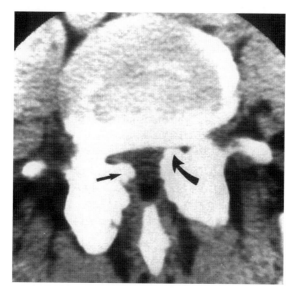

Plate 11   CT scan of elderly patient showing narrow spinal canal.

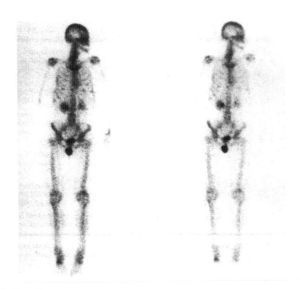

Plate 12 Normal bone scan.

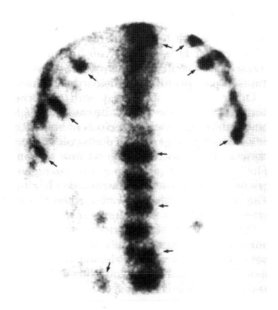

Plate 13 Abnormal bone scan showing metastatic deposits from prostate cancer.

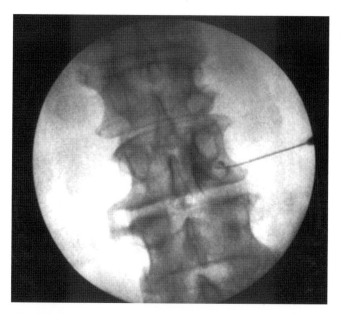

Plate 14   Lumbar nerve root block.

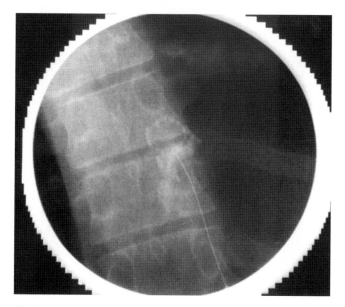

Plate 15   Thoracic facet joint injection.

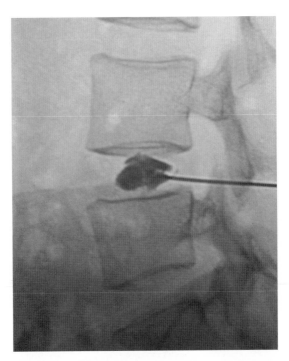

Plate 16   Normal disc appearance at L4-5.

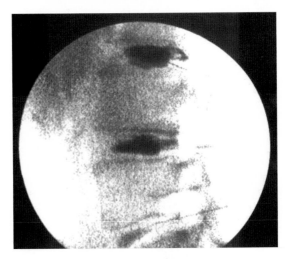

Plate 17   Three-level discography with posterior annular tears in the upper two levels.

be able to offer similar techniques for pain relief. In some districts, new structures within the health service are being established which offer a range of approaches that incorporate specialist GPs or doctors with recognized competency in the relief of severe and chronic musculoskeletal pain. The GP with special interest sometimes works in the community or is based in the hospital or part of a multi-professional team alongside physiotherapists, podiatrists, nurse practitioners and other paramedical professionals.

If the clinical picture is obvious and there are no concerns about other pathology causing the pain, there is really no need for an X-ray or a Magnetic Resonance Imaging (MRI) scan. However, this may vary between districts and, in some services, specialists are of the opinion that an MRI scan has to be obtained before invasive techniques such as epidurals or nerve root blocks can be given. This inevitably slows down the process of providing fast track pain relief.

Severe nerve root pain can be one of the more demoralizing experiences of back pain since some people are unable to obtain relief in any particular position or posture, and lose sleep night after night. This soon wears them down and they become rapidly depressed and hopeless. This category of patient needs special help in the form of adequate pain relief.

The current guidelines suggest that strong analgesics, such as opiates like morphine, should not be given in this context. This is a hangover from the days when prescription of opiates was less well regulated and repeat prescriptions for people with chronic pain were given, allowing them to become dependent on these narcotic substances. Every now and again, the dependent addictive personality would find it very difficult to relinquish morphine even when the pain was better controlled. However, these situations are

Q My doctor keeps telling me that it is 'nothing serious' but he hasn't got to suffer the pain. Surely something must be wrong if it is so painful and is not going away?

A Your doctor does not mean to belittle your problem but is simply trying to impress on you that severe prolonged pain from a trapped nerve does not imply a sinister disease such as cancer.

few and far between. Modern evidence on pain control shows that adequate pain relief, at whatever level is required, is the best method to prevent long-term disability. There really is little risk in giving strong opiate analgesics such as morphine for short-term use, that is to say up to two weeks for someone in severe pain.

Physiotherapists, osteopaths and chiropractors

Q **What is the best kind of manipulative therapist – a physiotherapist, osteopath or chiropractor?**

A Your doctor may be able to recommend someone who works closely with their practice or health centre who can provide some hands-on treatment and advice on exercise and rehabilitation. Most often, in the UK National Health Service (NHS), this would be a physiotherapist who is trained in musculoskeletal work. However, osteopaths and chiropractors are increasingly being used as alternative physical therapists who can provide a similar range of skills. All three of these practitioners will treat the same kind of patients and all have slightly different perspectives and treatment approaches. Essentially, however, there is more similarity than difference. For back pain that is not improving within a week or ten days, manipulation has been shown in many studies to speed recovery.

Manipulation

Manipulation of the spine, whether done by a physiotherapist, osteopath or chiropractor, is just as likely to be effective no matter which particular method is applied. Manipulation in the public mind may suggest obtaining a 'crack' or a 'click' or 'clunk' from a joint when a specific manual technique is applied as a short, sharp thrust. However, there are many techniques which do not require such vigorous mobilization, and which can be just as effective. These include Maitlands' mobilization, muscle energy technique, passive intervertebral movements, spontaneous release by positioning, strain–counterstrain, and so on. The principle behind all these techniques is to mobilize the joint that is stiff or stuck, and release the muscle spasm or tension that is helping bind it. There is good evidence that the audible 'click' produced by **gapping a joint** causes a reflex relaxation of the associated muscles, and this in itself can be beneficial.

gapping a joint
This describes a high velocity thrust type of manipulation creating separation of the joint surfaces for a moment. This may be accompanied by an audible click. It does not indicate a bone or disc being put back into place.

myth
Manipulation is putting something back into place.

fact
There is no evidence that the manipulation is achieving either reduction of a disc herniation or putting a bone back in place. This is a myth. There are some theories that the small pad of cartilage in the facet joint that acts as a space filler in the recess of a joint may become trapped, a bit like the torn cartilage in the knee causing a locked knee. Manipulation to 'gap' a facet joint may release this trapped pad, allowing restoration of normal gliding movement of the two articular surfaces.

There is research evidence that shows that range of motion does improve immediately following such manipulation, and this may help you on the road to recovery. There are some rumours that disc protrusion and prolapses cannot safely be manipulated. All experienced physical therapists from whatever persuasion are aware of the contraindications of manipulation. If there is a major threat to nerve roots or spinal cord tissue, they will not use techniques likely to cause risk. The potential risk, therefore, from manipulation of the spine is likely to come only from the unskilled therapist or practitioner who is not properly registered or certificated. Your doctor is only likely to recommend or refer you to a registered physical therapist who will be fully aware of the risks and benefits of manipulation and will take into account your previous medical history, age, bone strength and circulatory health.

my experience

I am a 29-year-old self-employed builder and I was recently in the middle of a job that I wanted to complete since bad weather had already caused delay and the houseowners were getting rather uptight. During this, I unfortunately strained my lower back while unloading some heavy blocks from a lorry. I called my general practice and got through to the triage nurse. She read out advice to me for acute back pain: 'keep as active as you can, don't lie down longer than you absolutely need to and don't worry, it's unlikely to be serious.' This advice was all very well but hardly applied to me. It didn't help me to do my job better because the pain would get worse over the day the more I tried to do. On the advice of my dad, also a builder, I went to see an osteopath who had a good reputation in my home town.

The osteopath listened to my story as I told him that I had been doing heavy manual work for 12 years. As well as working hard I explained that I also played football on the weekends. I told him that I drove round in an old truck with a very poor seat and was trying to run two or three jobs at the same time, each about 40 km apart. When the osteopath examined me, he told me the examination showed a 2-cm leg length deficit on the right, a slight scoliosis with a bend towards the right, also present on sitting, due apparently to an asymmetric pelvis. He said that my right leg muscles were slightly wasted, particularly the calf. The lumbar spine was restricted, I was tender at the lowest vertebral level (L5) and there were signs of sacroiliac strain with compensatory rotation.

So he treated me with manipulation of the sacroiliac joint on the left, specific high velocity thrust to the lowest lumbar vertebra (L5/S1) to 'gap' on the right and advised a 5-mm heel raise in the right shoe. He also advised a small wedge under my right buttock for sitting or driving as well as a lumbar wedge for support in the small of the back! He recommended a new seat for the truck and perhaps a new truck in the long run. I found it particularly helpful that the osteopath advised me on correct lifting and carrying techniques and suggested that I reduce my workload for the next three months by not taking on any more commitments.

I went to see him three more times over the next month, and he used manual techniques and recommended raising my right heel raise incrementally with a total build-up of 1 cm. He asked me to check with my parents whether there had been any suggestion of a viral illness in my childhood causing poliomyelitis. Apparently, this could explain my slightly smaller, weaker right leg. This turned out to be true! The osteopath then advised me to consider alternate recreational sports such as cycling or swimming since I tended to kick with my dominant left foot.

It is important to realize that manipulation is not the be all and end all on your road to recovery. It is simply an ancillary aid to get you back on your feet and active. Most of the hard work in terms of maintaining good posture, looking after the back and learning how to use the muscles properly to safeguard the back has to be done by you. Most well-trained physical therapists will not apply manipulation to the spine more than three or four times for one episode. Other rehabilitation work may need to be done in the course of treatment but one should be expecting improvement within the first two or three visits. If there is no improvement with this kind of approach, you should discuss this with your therapist and perhaps your doctor to consider other options. There is good evidence that manipulation works well for acute and chronic mechanical back and neck pain, including mid-back pain where there is no sign of nerve root pain or compression. However, there is no good evidence that it works any better than time and natural resolution for nerve root compression. Of course, there are always exceptions to this rule and sometimes one or two treatments are worth a try in the early stages because manipulation is a simple non-invasive treatment.

All the manual and rehabilitation approaches can be taken without resorting to any special investigations. If, after six to eight weeks, the problem is not improving and you are still not back to usual activity or work, then it is advised to meet and discuss the lack of progress with your doctor, the therapist or any other practitioner involved. This should happen automatically if you are already being treated by a multi-professional triage team, which is one of the new NHS structures. The GP with special interest in musculoskeletal disorders will ensure that there is adequate provision made to review any case that is not improving fairly quickly. At this point, there may be other factors delaying recovery. These are discussed in the earlier chapters and generally come under the heading of the 'yellow flags'. This refers to issues such as high levels of stress, anxiety, fear avoidance behaviour, depression and negative thinking. If these factors are identified, it is recommended that a psychologist becomes involved since the recovery may require a more holistic approach. If the doctor suspects more serious disease he or she will arrange blood tests, either an X-ray or bone scan and referral to a specialist.

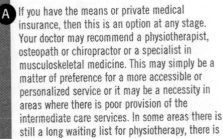

Q Should I consult someone privately?

A If you have the means or private medical insurance, then this is an option at any stage. Your doctor may recommend a physiotherapist, osteopath or chiropractor or a specialist in musculoskeletal medicine. This may simply be a matter of preference for a more accessible or personalized service or it may be a necessity in areas where there is poor provision of the intermediate care services. In some areas there is still a long waiting list for physiotherapy, there is

A no multi-professional team or doctor with special interest, and referral to a hospital specialist may involve a delay of many weeks or months. The private specialist would be able to provide most of the skills required in treating back pain under one roof, that is manipulation, trigger point injections or dry needling, epidural injection or nerve root block and, of course, an appropriate exercise prescription.

my experience

I am a 55-year-old businessman and I was involved in a rear-end motor vehicle accident resulting in neck ache and headache which had persisted for one month. I had been to see the GP, who prescribed painkillers and a soft collar. I was recommended by a friend to see a chiropractor who noticed generalized restricted movements, probably related to spondylosis of the cervical spine. He also noticed that I was tender and stiff at the joint between my second and third cervical vertebrae, C2/3 level, on both sides. He treated me with manipulation and postural exercises including active upper cervical neck retraction.

I had been quite shaken by the accident and had difficulty getting back in the driving seat due to an irrational fear of a further accident and repeat of the circumstances. I had been having nightmares about the accident, visualizing a large articulated truck descending on me from behind while stationary at the traffic lights. The anxiety this had provoked led to me losing my confidence and I would be the first to admit I was not functioning well at work. On return to work, which involved a certain amount of driving, I had a relapse of symptoms.

When the chiropractor re-examined me, he found evidence of diffuse muscle tension in the neck and across the shoulders. He treated this with trigger point needling (intramuscular stimulation) and recommended that I saw a psychologist to deal with the symptoms of **post-traumatic stress disorder**. I realized that I needed to deal with more than just the physical problem, and I was relieved that the chiropractor recommended this.

post-traumatic stress disorder

A psychological state arising from a fright or shock when a person perceives their survival has been threatened. This may follow any accident and bears no relation to the degree of injury actually sustained.

CHAPTER

6

Investigations and treatments

Still not improving?

In the UK, the boundary between primary care offered by the GP or physical therapist and secondary care available in the hospital has become less distinct. In order to improve services for musculoskeletal disorders, several initiatives to stem the epidemic of back pain (seen in the late 1980s and early 1990s) have been initiated. The government advisory group reporting on back pain in 1994 introduced the concept of triage by the general practitioner (GP). This report also stated clearly that most back pain could be treated at a primary care level without recourse to secondary care from specialists. However, if a patient was not improving within the first six to eight weeks, then referral should be made to an appropriately trained expert. This report indicated that in most circumstances this should not be the orthopaedic surgical department. This is because surgery is rarely undertaken for back pain and that the long wait for an orthopaedic opinion, which in itself tends to create chronicity, would all too often result in the anticipated opinion – 'surgery is not indicated, what you need is more physiotherapy'. Equally inappropriate is referral to a rheumatology specialist whose primary role is to diagnose and manage inflammatory disease of the joints. In the vast majority of cases, this does not apply to the spine and therefore most rheumatologists will be less prepared to deal with the common problem of back pain than a specialist physiotherapist, a GP with special interest or a musculoskeletal or sports physician.

Which specialist is ideal?

In the early 1990s, three of the eight districts visited by the UK government working party found that orthopaedic/musculoskeletal physicians were already in post providing a service for back pain sufferers, although usually from a secondary care base, i.e. in hospital. The initiatives put forward soon after this report have been taken up in some areas. These include a musculoskeletal service either based in the community, headed by a GP with special interest, together with a team of physical therapists, or a hospital-based service with input from orthopaedics, rheumatology, the pain service, the musculoskeletal physician (in some areas) and specifically skilled physiotherapists. Ideally, this multi-professional team should include a clinical psychologist. However, in many areas, this is not available. As a result there is a huge variation in the service level provided for back pain across the UK. In one area there may be hospital-based specialists in musculoskeletal medicine working as part of a team with physiotherapists and podiatrists, and also going out to work in the community with GPs. This service would also be involved in training GPs to develop special skills in triage and management of back pain. In another area, the orthopaedic department may have appointed a specialist physiotherapist to perform triage and, in some instances, initiate investigations where appropriate and then either treat or arrange appropriate referral to the relevant specialist. Other options available include primary care teams employing musculoskeletal physicians and specialist physiotherapists directly to offer a service which is community based. Ideally, these doctors and specialist practitioners would also be working part-time in the hospital so that a patient's journey through the various levels of care would appear to be seamless. Those patients with severe back pain or nerve root pain would have rapid access to a pain relief service provided either by the musculoskeletal physician or pain specialist in the hospital. If the back sufferer is becoming chronically disabled and the existence of psychosocial factors delaying recovery has been identified, a clinical psychologist should be involved as part of the team early on.

The distinction between primary care and secondary care is somewhat blurred since some of these services exist in what is now termed an 'intermediate level of care' or interface clinic provided between the hospital and GP. The term 'specialist' therefore may refer to a wide range of practitioners from the extended scope practitioner (specialist physiotherapist) to the musculoskeletal physician, pain specialist, rheumatologist or orthopaedic surgeon.

To make it easier we will refer to a 'generic specialist' whose post-graduate training may vary considerably from surgical training to manual therapy, rehabilitation or injection techniques. It would seem logical for this generic specialist to be multi-skilled, however, it is unlikely that any such specialist would be able to acquire all the skills of surgical training and the various forms of medical and rehabilitation treatment. Therefore, the logical division must occur between surgery and non-surgical treatment. Since most patients do not require surgery, it would seem that this generic specialist should ideally be skilled at a higher level than the GP and physiotherapist in terms of being able to provide the entire range of non-surgical medical treatment. This includes manipulation, rehabilitation principles, soft tissue, trigger point and spinal injections together with a good understanding of the psychologist's approach to managing chronic pain and disability. At the present time, this combination of skills is most likely to be found in the musculoskeletal physician. However, these are relatively few in number, acquiring their training through a variety of different post-graduate routes. There is no doubt that many more need to be trained to provide an equitable service across the country.

If your condition has not improved as a result of care from your general practitioner and physiotherapy in approximately eight weeks, or less if you have been experiencing severe nerve root pain, you should have access to this 'generic specialist' for further advice and treatment.

my experience

I am a 45-year-old lady and, admittedly, rather overweight. I work as a care attendant in a local nursing home. Over the last few years I have had increasing episodes of low back pain, each time resulting in my back feeling twisted, and people have remarked that I look lopsided during these acute attacks. I was being managed by my GP and had already had a course of physiotherapy and seen an osteopath a couple of times for each acute episode. However, I was becoming concerned because the attacks were happening several times a year and, after the last attack, I had lost two

fact
Despite the surge in research in recent years there are still many gaps in knowledge and understanding of the causes of back pain. The humble expert is quick to admit this.

months from work. My GP referred me to a multi-professional triage team working at the local hospital trust. There, I saw an extended scope physiotherapist who recommended stabilization training for my low back.

After two or three months I had a further episode and was then referred to see the musculoskeletal doctor who worked as part of the multi-professional team. He prescribed a course of ligament sclerosant injections (prolotherapy) aimed at the lower lumbar L4/5 and L5/S1 spinal ligaments. He reviewed me three months later having advised me to keep up the muscle training exercises to maintain core stability. Brilliantly, I have since had no further episodes and now feel much more positive about my future prospects for work.

The specialist appointment

If you have back pain that has been going on for more than six to eight weeks or you are suffering from chronic recurrent back pain and are still off work, then obviously you require a reasonable amount of time for consultation, examination and advice with a specialist. Most specialists allow at least half an hour for seeing a new patient since any attempt to get to grips with a complex multifactorial problem such as chronic back pain requires adequate time allocation. A patient presenting at this stage may have a number of concerns and worries about the cause of their back pain: whether it will get better, their future job prospects, whether or not they need surgery, to name just a few. The specialist should allow the sufferer the time to talk and to give a full account of their symptoms and their concerns in an initial interview. Following the interview, the specialist will examine the patient with a basic orthopaedic examination, including assessment of range of motion of the back and limb joints with palpation for tenderness. If nerve root symptoms or signs are present, he or she will also be able to carry out a full examination of the nervous system assessing signs of loss of sensation, weakness of muscles and loss of reflex. Any symptoms pertaining to impairment of bladder or bowel function will require a more detailed examination of sphincter tone and sensation around the perineum. In addition to the basic aspects of examination, the specialist should ideally be able to assess the spinal joints, pelvis and soft tissues for signs of dysfunction. This requires the acquisition of **palpatory skills** of the kind that osteopaths, manipulating physiotherapists, chiropractors and musculoskeletal physicians learn and apply routinely. This is vital because the vast majority of back pain sufferers, even at this stage, will be suffering predominantly from various manifestations of spinal dysfunction rather than pathology identified by imaging and laboratory tests.

palpatory skills
The ability to detect, purely by touch and passive movements, subtle changes in the soft tissues and joint play.

After the examination, the specialist will provide enough time to sit down and talk to a patient about his or her view of the problem and, where appropriate, attempt to allay any fears and concerns.

How useful is an X-ray?

A plain X-ray of the lumbar spine used to be recommended for all back sufferers with pain that had endured for more than eight weeks. However, it has been increasingly recognized that the positive yield from these images of the spine, which involve ionizing radiation, is relatively low. The images shown in the Plate section identify the following:

1 Spondylolisthesis (Plate 1)
2 Spondylolysis (Plate 2)
3 Degenerative spondylolisthesis
4 Bony anomaly (Plate 6)
5 Vertebral compression fracture (Plate 5).

The first four of the above conditions can be found fairly commonly among people without back pain. It is difficult to relate these changes found on X-ray with the actual symptoms that you are suffering unless there is severe degeneration of a disc at one level or a marked forward slip, i.e. more than Grade 2 (50 per cent of the vertebra or more overlaps the one below). Only in the fifth example, vertebral compression fracture, is X-ray likely to be of any direct clinical utility. Therefore, plain X-rays are performed relatively rarely these days other than to reassure a worried patient. Far too often patients may be informed of so-called abnormal findings on an X-ray which, rather than serving to reassure them, are misinterpreted and tend to compound the anxiety. The significance of these findings has to be explained very carefully to avoid misconceptions.

Even chiropractors who traditionally have X-rayed every patient who walks into their office have now ceased doing X-rays for most of their back pain patients. The key point is that X-rays only show the bones and the spaces between the bones. Most back problems are not caused directly by problems with the bones unless there is compression or collapse or the presence of some gross pathology in the bone itself. X-rays are not useful for looking at small alterations in the positions of bones since they show a two-dimensional view, and exact bony position can only be determined using a three-dimensional view. There is still a vogue for assessing mobility of certain regions of the spine by looking at the movement of the vertebrae and how they vary between positions of extreme flexion and extension. This can be useful in the rare instance of diagnosing the movements between the atlas and axis (the top two vertebrae) in rheumatoid patients, but otherwise there is such wide variability in the translational mobility of vertebrae that most of the time such 'functional views' are not useful.

The concept of **lumbar instability** is a clinical one rather than one that can be shown through radiological (X-ray) assessment. This clinical concept refers more to 'micro' movements of the bone, changing patterns of stress and strain in the soft tissues provoking pain. Spondylolisthesis, where one bone slips forward or occasionally backward on another, is not usually unstable in a mechanical sense although of course there are increased stresses, both on the adjacent disc and the associated facet joints, which may provoke pain syndromes.

> **lumbar instability**
> A controversial term which, in the context used here, refers only to the patient's subjective experience of their problem and the specialist's hypothetical explanation. It does not mean that there are any visible excessive movements of one vertebra on another.

How useful is an MRI scan?

Magnetic Resonance Imaging (MRI) is undoubtedly the most sensitive form of imaging for screening for more serious pathology in the spine. It displays the state of the discs, the presence of protrusions or prolapses, the spinal cord and nerve roots, the facet joints and ligamentum flavum (yellow ligament), blood vessels and the muscles and larger ligaments. This amount of detail needs to be interpreted carefully.

Most often an MRI scan (see Plate 7) only needs to be done to exclude more serious pathology or to confirm the presence of a suspected disc prolapse and the level at which it is situated in order to plan appropriate invasive treatment, for example, nerve root block under X-ray control or surgery in the form of removal of the disc fragment. However, MRI is increasingly used as a response to the demands from the back sufferer for a specific diagnosis. It is already clear that plain X-rays cannot help with diagnosis or management in a vast majority of back pain problems. This is true to a lesser extent with MRI scanning. The problem is that in many ways it is too sensitive an instrument; structural abnormalities, mainly to do with the state of disc degeneration, bulges and protrusions will show up commonly in people who do not have back pain – some of whom have never had back pain. Approximately 35 per cent of a normal, non-suffering population shows these abnormalities. Therefore, if similar findings appear in somebody with back pain, it is difficult to be certain of how the findings correlate directly with the patient's symptoms and source of pain. However, the main advantage of MRI scanning is that there is no known risk or harm to the patient. It is a picture obtained by placing the body in a tube surrounded by large coils which generate a high strength magnetic field. This affects the hydrogen atoms in the water of the body (the body is approximately 80 per cent water), and they are oriented along the lines of the magnetic field. A radio-frequency signal is then sent into the tissues, and the resulting discharge is identified and processed as images which can be collected as slices through the body at any angle to build up a three-dimensional picture. In this way, the changes in the water content can reflect the changes in the tissue such as inflammation, swelling, bleeding, etc. MRI scanning is not as sensitive for identifying small fractures in the bones or alterations in the bone shape as the earlier technology of Computerized Axial Tomography, a sophisticated X-ray technique commonly known as a CT scan.

my experience

I am a 72-year-old retired gentleman and I enjoy much of my time fishing and gardening. I like to walk down to the social club, about 4 km, two evenings a week to catch up on the news with my ex-work mates. However, over the last year, I found that my legs were becoming increasingly heavy, like lead, after a short distance and I sometimes had to sit down on the way. Although I had always smoked a bit, I didn't get puffed and I felt generally fit. My walking distance reduced to 180 m because of this and I was beginning to fear a life of social isolation. I was beginning to feel my age for the first time in my life.

On the advice of one of my friends, I went to see a sports therapist who gave me massage on four occasions and said that I had arthritis in my knees. This had made no difference, so I consulted my GP who examined me carefully, listened to my heart and checked my blood pressure. She felt for the pulses in my legs and feet. She told me that my circulation was good despite my tobacco habit and that I did have stiff, arthritic knees but that after 60 years' smoking, perhaps now was the time to give up. I asked what difference it would make to my legs. She couldn't promise it would definitely make a difference and offered to do a blood test to check for thyroid problems and anaemia. She also arranged a chest X-ray to rule out lung cancer. All these tests were normal so I asked if I could have a second opinion. She sent me to the local musculoskeletal doctor who worked part-time in orthopaedics and part-time in the community for the primary care trust.

The doctor saw me within a few weeks and listened carefully to my account. He noticed stiff movements of the spine, apparently not unusual for my age, osteoarthritis of the knees and normal pulses in the legs and feet. He arranged to take me outside and watch me walking. As usual, at about 140 m, I started to shuffle, the right foot dropping a little. The doctor could see that my gait became slow and unsteady. On return, the specialist asked me whether I could walk further when going up hill. I said that the odd thing was when I went to the supermarket to shop with my wife I could push the trolley around the aisles for hours if I had to. The specialist ordered an MRI scan promptly which showed me the problem — narrowing of the spinal canal at two levels in the lumbar region at the third and fourth vertebrae, L3/4 and the fourth and fifth vertebrae, L4/5. The musculoskeletal doctor discussed options in management which included walking with a stick to remain slightly forwards, an epidural steroid injection or referral for surgery. I opted for the injection first which gave me six months' relief.

 So where is the pain coming from?

 State of the art imaging falls far short of telling you this information. It only shows changes in structure or inflammatory reactions. It does not light up the site of pain production unfortunately.

A scan that is normal for your age can be very reassuring, but unfortunately there is a tendency for many doctors and specialists to describe the 'normal abnormalities' to a patient in terms of degeneration, disc bulge, facet joint osteoarthritis, which, rather than serving to reassure a patient, worries them. There is also a tendency to over-interpret these changes, implying that they are a cause of the patient's pain. As fascinating as it may be to look at these beautiful images of the interior of the spine, most often our state of the art imaging does not answer the question, 'Where is the back pain coming from?' However, despite these misconceptions, an MRI scan is a huge improvement on the very limited investigations that used to be available to identify disc prolapse (see Plates 8 and 9) and spinal cord tumour or other causes of nerve root compression.

MRI scanning is sensitive enough to detect early signs of stress in the bone before an actual fracture occurs, as in the junior athlete's pars interarticularis stress reaction (see Chapter 4, page 69). It will also identify the inflammatory changes in the bones around the sacroiliac joint in ankylosing spondylitis (see Chapter 4, page 64) and other forms of inflammatory disease of the pelvis and spine. Sometimes unexpected injuries crop up such as tears in the deep muscles of the spine although these are rare. Specialists will vary in their threshold for ordering an MRI scan, but in some cases this has replaced the use of a plain X-ray as the initial investigation for back pain which is at a risk of becoming chronic at the six to eight week stage. If laboratory blood tests have not been done by your doctor, then the specialist may consider ordering a full blood count, red cell sedimentation rate (ESR) or plasma viscosity test, calcium phosphate, alkaline phosphatase, vitamin D levels, electrophoretic strip looking for plasma proteins (myeloma), acid phosphatase (prostate cancer screen), prostate specific antigen (PSA), uric acid (gout), and rheumatoid factor tests. These tests would be among the ones most commonly ordered to screen for disease affecting the spine. The sensitivity of the ESR, the sedimentation rate of the red cells, is reasonably good for detecting serious pathology. None of these tests is absolutely foolproof, and the use and interpretation of them is a matter for your specialist's clinical judgement.

CT scan

The CT (Computerized axial Tomography) scan is a slightly older technology than MRI but is excellent at identifying the detailed state of the bones. This is because images can be built up in slices to produce a three-dimensional impression of the shape of the bone, its position, and the presence of any internal fractures or defects (see Plates 10 and 11). A CT scan also shows the disc tissue, but nerves are not easily identified. An advantage to using a CT scan is when a patient cannot enter into a high magnetic field, for example, when they have an implanted pacemaker.

Furthermore, the presence of metalware, which may have been used for previous back surgery, distorts the images obtained by MRI whereas those obtained by CT scanning remain clear. A CT scan is also useful for picking up changes in the bone at an earlier stage in the disease process than could be identified with X-ray. Subtle changes in the underlying bone present in the margins of an osteoarthritic joint would not show up on plain X-rays until there has been approximately a 40 per cent change in structure.

Bone scan

The radioisotope bone scan employs the use of a radioactive tracer chemical injected into a vein, which then circulates through the body and is taken up particularly by the bones (see Plate 12).

Two or three hours later, emissions from this radioactive chemical can be detected from the bone, particularly where there are highly active bone-producing cells. This is used to detect areas where there has been a fracture or some other cause for excessive reaction of the bone such as the presence of tumours and metastatic deposits (see Plate 13).

A bone scan is a way of surveying the whole skeleton and obtaining a view of areas of abnormal activity, usually termed 'hot spots'. However, the change in activity has to be quite intense before one can be certain a genuine problem is being identified since wear and tear and degeneration of the joints do produce a less intense hot spot. A bone scan can also be used to detect reduced bone activity (regional ostoporosis) which can occur in a patchy distribution when there is disturbance of the sympathetic nervous system. These conditions are termed 'complex regional pain syndromes' (reflex sympathetic dystrophy), see Chapter 8, page 133.

Nerve conduction studies

These tests are most commonly requested by specialists when they are considering causes for nerve root disturbance other than compression due to disc protrusion. The tests are done by a neurophysiologist who puts fine needles in various muscles and uses small electrical signals to determine whether a nerve is functioning or not. The presence of electrical activity detected in the muscles can also help with defining the kind of nerve damage that has occurred, its severity and detecting other diseases of the neuromuscular system. Nerve conduction studies are not required

Q **Why hasn't my specialist ordered more investigations?**

A You may think that the specialist's main role is to decide whether or not further investigations need to be done, but most of the time with back pain there is very little requirement for investigation. It is mainly a question of using clinical experience and judgement to decide the best way to manage a problem in order to prevent it becoming chronic. The interpretation of any tests and the explanation to the patient are the most important aspects of specialist care together with identification of the anxieties and health beliefs of the patient.

very often in the detection of back pain and its related nerve root problems except when more than one nerve root has been involved and the diagnosis is uncertain.

Treatments

The specialist should ideally be able to provide treatments that give good pain relief for nerve root pain without long delays. Due to the fact that prolonged pain and sleepless nights can lead to demoralization and depression in some individuals, efficient and effective action is paramount.

Epidural steroid injection

The most widely used intervention for acute disc prolapse with nerve root involvement is the epidural (into the space around the dura mater of the spine) steroid injection. This can be given via the caudal route (see Figure 6.1), just above the tail bone, where there is a natural opening at the base of the sacrum, or between the lumbar vertebrae close to the affected level of disc prolapse.

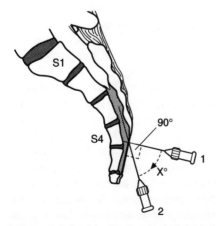

Figure 6.1 Caudal epidural route of administration.

Either route may be effective but there is no guarantee that the medication administered will spread to the main site of irritation, which is usually at the front of the spinal canal where the disc is bulging back towards the nerve. At present, most of these treatments are done without the benefit of X-ray control and the use of contrast medium. Contrast medium is a dye, visible on X-ray screening (fluoroscopy), that is injected so that its flow and distribution can be observed. Furthermore, the use of contrast medium ensures that the operator is not injecting the medicine into a small vein, which would simply remove the medicine from the appropriate treatment area into the general circulation. The rather variable response to epidural injections is probably a combination of the following two factors:

1 The injection is usually done 'blind' without the benefit of **fluoroscopic control**
2 There is no contrast medium to determine spread and flow of the injected material.

However, whichever route is used, epidural injection can be an effective way of relieving the pain of inflammation caused by the enzymes from a degenerating disc irritating the nerve root. It has been shown that these enzymes actually damage the nerve root and that the use of corticosteroid has a beneficial, anatagonistic effect on the enzymes.

The epidural injection is usually given either in a safe outpatient setting such as a treatment room or procedure room, or in a day surgery unit. There is quite a wide variation in the amount of local anaesthetic that is mixed with the corticosteroid and, in many outpatient settings, physicians use normal saline since it is the corticosteroid which is the active ingredient. The local anaesthetic merely provides extra volume and may be useful to give direct feedback about whether the target area has

fluoroscopic control
The use of X-ray guidance to direct needles or other instruments accurately to the anatomical target.

myth
Epidurals are dangerous and can cause permanent scarring.

fact
A small minority of patients are prone to develop scarring in the spinal canal for a variety of reasons, but there is no evidence that epidurals play a part in this.

been reached – numbness and reduction of pain will occur much quicker with the use of local anaesthetic. This technique is relatively safe, providing certain basic guidelines are adhered to:

✧ The operator must be adequately trained and competent for the technique
✧ An aseptic or no-touch technique must be used to avoid infection
✧ The treatment should be given in a clean and sterile environment
✧ The use of resuscitation facilities in the event of complications should be to hand.

Complications from this injection are very rare but may include infection, bleeding, allergy, and toxicity from the use of excessive quantities of local anaesthetic which have been taken up by other tissues such as the brain and heart.

Nerve root block

A more specific and targeted treatment using smaller doses of local anaesthetic and corticosteroid may be given to the nerve root which is directly under compression or irritated by the disc prolapse. This usually necessitates MRI scanning in advance of the intervention in order to identify how and where the nerve root is being irritated. A small dose is delivered at the end of a needle which is placed by direct fluoroscopic screening close to the nerve. A contrast medium (dye) is used first to identify good flow around the nerve (see Plate 14) before a small dose of the medication is administered. The same safety and complication factors apply as in epidurals.

> **myth**
> Treatments to numb the pain allow one to continue damaging the spine without knowing.

> **fact**
> Reducing inflammation is one way of allowing the nerve root to recover and for normal motion to ensue. No treatment can take all the pain away, so there is no risk of harm.

Facet joint injections

The diagnosis of facet joint pain is not an easy one to make. Because the facet joints are situated at the back of the spine and bear increased load on extension, particularly combined with rotation, it seems logical that the pain caused by these movements might be due to the facet joints. Furthermore, tenderness directly over these joints is quite commonly found in mechanical back pain. However, research has shown that there are no simple clinical tests that will diagnose pain arising from these joints with any reliability. Recent research has shown that mechanical back pain in the over-65 age group brought on by upright activity and relieved by sitting or lying down, which is not aggravated by any specific active lumbar movement, are the only symptoms and physical signs which suggest facet joint pain. In order to prove this, however, local anaesthetic blocking of the small nerves supplying the joint or injection into the joints must be done – preferably on two separate occasions to confirm these joints are painful. In practice, a small dose of corticosteroid with local anaesthetic is injected into the facet joint (see Plate 15) and followed up with appropriate exercises to reduce the strain on these structures. In younger patients this may settle a prolonged episode due to an acute strain. Nevertheless, in worn joints that are arthritic, as in the elderly, the pain does tend to return within a few weeks or months.

Facet denervation

If the pain returns soon after facet joint injection, facet denervation can be used to obtain more prolonged relief. A small heat probe is applied to the small branch that innervates the joint for 60–90 seconds to deactivate the nerve. This treatment is commonly performed in pain clinics but some other specialists also offer it. Facet joint pain seems to account for approximately 15 per cent of chronic mechanical back pain in younger patients, rising to 40 per cent in the elderly. In the neck, however, the predominance of facet joint pain is higher, probably because these joints are larger in relation to the intervertebral disc joint and are prone to strain in whiplash-type injury. In whiplash situations, these joints may account for up to 50 per cent of patients with chronic neck pain. Occasionally these joints may become a problem in the thoracic spine, and injections or denervation may be applied to this region in the same way. Such treatment is always done under X-ray control to confirm accurate placement of the needle, and is usually carried out either on an outpatient basis or as a minor day case procedure in the appropriate setting.

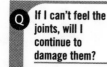

 If I can't feel the joints, will I continue to damage them?

Facet denervation does not eliminate the entire nerve supply to the joint, so the joint continues to function normally.

Prolotherapy

The term 'prolotherapy' is short for fibroproliferative therapy which literally means the provocation of new fibrous tissue formation for treatment and is achieved by the injection of an irritant solution, usually a mixture of a small amount of phenol with concentrated dextrose and glycerine (mixed with local anaesthetic), into each end of the ligament that connects two bones. Prolotherapy treats ligamentous pain and laxity. This treatment has been available for 50 years and was first developed in North America by a surgeon who was tending to patients who had suffered injury from industrial or motor-vehicle accidents. He found that the ligaments – principally the interspinous ligaments, facet joint capsules, the ligaments of the pelvis and those linking the last two lumbar vertebrae, L4 and L5 with the ilium – were prone to strain and sometimes relaxation, i.e. overstretch leading to loss of the mechanical integrity of the joint as a whole. Sometimes the pain comes from the ligaments themselves which are richly innervated (supplied) with nerve endings, at other times from the associated joint structures controlled or restrained by these ligaments.

Selection of patients for this procedure is difficult, largely because there is little established agreement as to the optimum clinical features which would predict a good result from these injections. The studies that have been done have selected patients with pain provoked by prolonged static posture, either sitting or standing, or in those patients whose case history suggests minor degrees of instability, for example, the back frequently 'goes out'.

Perhaps the most recognizable syndrome is the female patient whose ligaments have relaxed during pregnancy to allow childbirth, but have failed to strengthen and tighten in the subsequent six months. These mothers also have to bear quite a lot of everyday stress and strain on their back in the care of their young baby, which in turn takes its toll. If the sufferer also tends towards ligamentous laxity, commonly termed '**hypermobility**', then the ligaments may simply be too loose to allow proper control and support from the pelvis. These mothers report frequent episodes of pain associated with the sacroiliac joint, on one side or the other, or sometimes both, which can be quite disabling.

hypermobility
Refers to joints which have more than average flexibility due to ligamentous laxity.

The other category of patient that often responds well to prolotherapy is those with minor degrees of spondylolisthesis, where one vertebra slips slightly forward on the other. This may cause mechanical pain due to compression on the facet joints, disturbance of disc mechanics in the adjacent joint and overstretch of the associated ligaments. However, the vast majority of patients selected for this procedure tend to have what is commonly termed 'mechanical back syndrome' which has not responded to the appropriate course of rehabilitation exercises, and evidence of hypermobile vertebral segments or sacroiliac joints. Specialists practising this particular form of treatment tend to come from a background of osteopathy or musculoskeletal medicine training where clinical palpation skills are relatively high and familiarity with various forms of mechanical back pain has been developed through long experience.

The small dose of sclerosant mixture, which is actually a sclerosant licensed for use in the treatment of varicose veins, is mixed with an equal amount of local anaesthetic and injected into the supra and interspinous ligaments as well as other involved ligaments which can be approached safely from the back. Half a millilitre of the mixture is injected into each ligamentous attachment in up to 16 or 20 places (see Figure 6.2 on page 112). This treatment is quite uncomfortable and the patient is usually relaxed with sedation or is given analgesic gas mixture to breathe to reduce the discomfort of the procedure. The ligaments react with an inflammatory response over the next couple of days, which makes the back stiff and sore and then, gradually, with repeated stimulation by further injection therapy given at weekly intervals on three to six occasions, the process of fibrosis restores ligamentous integrity and reduces the mechanical pain and instability. Sometimes the benefit does not emerge until three to six months after the course of treatment. Once established, the benefit may last for several years before requiring a booster treatment. It has not been clearly established whether this treatment also addresses faults due to tears within a disc substance itself, causing mechanical dysfunction of the whole intervertebral joint. Nevertheless, it is quite likely that this treatment may address the less severe cases of pain arising from internal disc disruption.

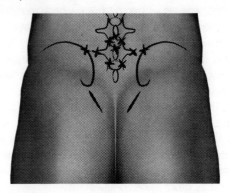

Figure 6.2 Surface marking of target points for injection.

> **myth**
> Prolotherapy is dangerous and has caused paralysis and death.

> **fact**
> There were a few cases reported of this happening in the early 1960s when a more toxic sclerosant was inadvertently injected into the spinal canal by untrained operators. No such event has occurred in the last 40 years with the use of a safe sclerosant solution in properly trained hands.

Discogenic pain and its management

If a specialist has been able to exclude significant disc prolapse with nerve root irritation or compression and there was no evidence of any other serious pathology affecting the spine, a proportion of patients with chronic mechanical back pain – approximately 40 per cent shown in one study – have pain arising from internal disc tears. Unfortunately, this diagnosis cannot be established from any imaging technique, including MRI. These images may suggest that certain discs are more liable to be the source of pain than others by their state of degeneration but it can only be proven by provocation discography (see Plate 16). Some specialists will undertake this procedure, under X-ray control, on patients with significant impairment of function and who have not responded to the standard rehabilitation measures over some months. If the pain and disability warrant this next step, the specialist will inject a small amount of contrast medium (dye) into selected discs one at a time to see if the patient's typical pain is reproduced with this form of pressurization. At the same time, using real time screening, tears through the annulus (the outer fibrous ring of the disc) can be identified. A significant tear to the periphery of the disc combined with reproduction of concordant pain (the exact pain the patient is suffering), is a positive finding. Not every specialist who works with spine patients believes in the value of this way of diagnosing discogenic pain. However, it has been used for several decades and has become increasingly popular, particularly for surgeons wishing to identify the painful disc level that may require surgical fusion.

my experience

I am a slim, active woman of 25, and I was very surprised to be a sufferer of lower lumbar and upper pelvic pain on and off for the last four years. The pain would sometimes be felt in the left buttock and at other times in the right buttock and would interfere in my ability to walk and stride out. Occasionally it would hurt with bending and lifting. I also felt that during these episodes my lower back was generally stiff, particularly in the morning. I had been seeing a chiropractor for some time and initially seemed to respond quite well to chiropractic adjustments.

However, for the last year this simply had not worked and so I consulted my GP. He noted the history and location of pain, and in particular the comment about the aching and stiffness in the lumbar and pelvic region first thing in the morning. Yet he found my back to be generally very mobile. He referred me to the local musculoskeletal specialist for a further opinion.

When I saw the specialist and told him my story, he examined me carefully, looking for signs of any limb length difference and evidence of hypermobility (lax joints). He performed ligamentous stress tests of the sacroiliac joints and found three out of the five of these tests to be positive. There was no evidence of any nerve root involvement or mechanical problem in the lumbar region. He put me on a ten-day course of anti-inflammatory medication which seemed to relieve my problem considerably. This led him to believe that I may be suffering from a form of inflammatory spine disease. He arranged an MRI scan which showed the presence of oedema (fluid) in the bones adjacent to the sacroiliac joints on both sides. He then explained to me that I had an inflammatory disorder of the spine called 'sacroiliitis' and arranged further blood tests which helped to confirm this diagnosis. He advised me on mobility exercises and the use of non-steroidal anti-inflammatory medication on a long-term basis. I was at last satisfied that I had an explanation for my ongoing symptoms and a strategy for managing it.

Chronic discogenic pain

A number of new treatments have been introduced since the mid-1990s to avoid the rather radical step of fusing two vertebrae together after removal of the entire disc. These techniques usually involve insertion of a fine catheter into the disc to heat the periphery of the annulus, where the pain fibres lie, to desensitize or denervate the disc (IDET – Intradiscal Electrothermal Therapy). It is also claimed that this may change the nature of the collagen structure causing some retraction and thickening, although this has not been proven. Other techniques are used – laser or plasma coblation (nucleoplasty) – to remove damaged disc material or to decompress the disc from within. There are also new techniques using radio-frequency current as an alternative way of providing direct heating. Although some of these techniques have certainly shown promise in earlier studies, the final proof of their long-term effectiveness still remains to be shown. Nevertheless, many patients will prefer a trial of this minimally invasive procedure to treat their chronic back pain rather than face the prospect of fusion (see Chapter 7, page 127).

The threshold for initiating minimally invasive interventions can vary enormously from one specialist to another, depending on their particular beliefs and persuasions. There are so many options available to the patient with chronic back pain at present, that the specialist will often consider a patient's values and beliefs about their pain rather than the specialist's preference.

> **Q** **My specialist has tried everything to get to the source of pain but nothing has had any lasting effect. Where do I go next?**
>
> **A** In about 25 per cent of patients with chronic back pain it is not possible to identify the source or, having done so, there is no single effective solution, hence the need for a pain management approach.

Medication

Although most of the simple pain medications and anti-inflammatory drugs may have been tried by your doctor in primary care, there are other more powerful or long-term medications that may be recommended by the specialist.

In the elderly, if osteoporosis has been diagnosed resulting in loss of height and increasingly bent posture (kyphosis), and particularly if a compression fracture has occurred, improvement of diet and supplementation with calcium and vitamin D would certainly be recommended. Specific hormones affecting bone metabolism called the 'bisphosphonates' will also be commenced and continued for some years to help build up the bones' mineralization. These drugs have been shown to reduce the incidence of further fracture whether in the spine or hip.

For those patients in whom an inflammatory condition has been diagnosed, such as sacroiliitis or ankylosing spondylitis, non-steroidal anti-inflammatory drugs such as ibuprofen will be commenced for long-term medication. It is rare for a patient to be put on oral steroids such as prednisolone purely for back pain since the long-term effect of this is to cause demineralization and osteoporosis.

However, there are some inflammatory conditions such as polymyalgia rheumatica, which cause pain around the shoulder and hip girdles, that do respond very well to oral steroid medication. The specialist will aim to commence the dose at a fairly high level to control symptoms and then gradually reduce to the minimum dose possible to maintain control of the condition. Bisphosphonates are usually considered in this event to preserve bone strength.

Pain control

For those people who are facing a life of chronic pain due to their back, Chapter 8 gives guidance on how to cope with the pain.

Other medications which may be offered by any of the doctors you encounter on your journey will include muscle relaxants, although they have only been shown to help in the acute spasms of short-term episodes. Tramadol and other synthetic opioids are thought to be less addictive than the opiate group of drugs, but they are not quite as strong. Dihydrocodeine and opiate drugs tend to have side effects, both in the short term (such as constipation), and in the long term (such as loss of motivation, sleepiness and impairment of cognitive function, reducing concentration). Further discussion on the use of these drugs can be found in Chapter 7.

Trigger point injections

Treating tense muscles anywhere in the back, neck or buttock, especially if there is trigger point formation, can be rewarding. Nevertheless, it should be explained that most back pain, other than prolonged postural strain fatiguing the muscles, is not due primarily to muscle injury. Referred pain from any of the structures in the spine is often accompanied by muscle tension and tenderness of these muscles. If this persists for more than a few weeks, the muscles themselves start to behave abnormally, developing taut bands and hyperactive foci called 'trigger points'. These can be treated by massage, pressure inhibition, ultrasound and other modalities offered by the physical therapist.

A trigger point is painful and refers pain to distant sites. The localized area of tension reduces the blood flow to the muscle which can then cause further pain due to the starvation of oxygen and the build-up of metabolites (products of inflammatory cell metabolism). This further pain caused by 'ischaemia' feeds back through the spinal reflex system to provoke more tension in response to the pain. This vicious circle can be interrupted in a variety of ways, but the underlying causes must also be addressed to achieve any lasting benefit. More difficult trigger points will often settle well with dry needling – the insertion of acupuncture needles into the tight bands or trigger points. If this is too painful for the patient to tolerate, then an alternative is the injection of a small amount of local anesthetic into the trigger point to break the vicious circle (see Figure 6.3 on page 118).

The specialist may utilize some of these techniques himself, particularly if working in a pain clinic or as a musculoskeletal physician. He or she may choose to refer the patient to somebody experienced in the technique of intramuscular stimulation or Western acupuncture.

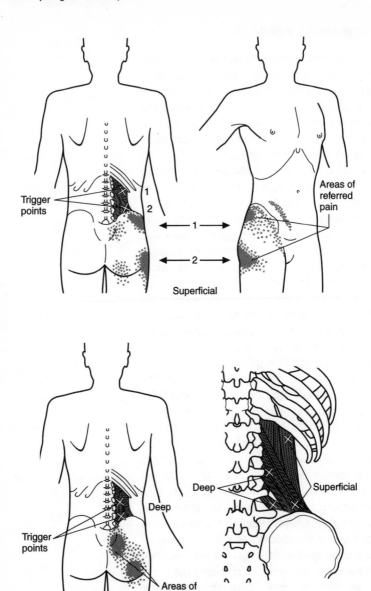

Figure 6.3 Myofascial pain syndrome in back muscles.

Sacroiliac joint pain

Specialists are divided in opinion about the frequency of the sacroiliac joint as a cause of common mechanical back pain, but it has been established in one study that this joint may account for up to 13 per cent of chronic back pain sufferers. Direct injection into the joint under X-ray control with local anaesthetic and steroid may settle the pain for a while and render a patient pain-free.

If the pain results from an inflammatory disorder, it is likely that the pain will return. If the pain is caused by mechanical dysfunction, once again the pain is likely to return unless the mechanical factors are addressed. These mechanical factors may be: hypermobility, in which case prolotherapy is an option; muscle imbalance, which requires appropriate physiotherapy; leg length difference, which requires a built-up shoe; or faulty techniques in sports or athletics. Some patients develop chronic sacroiliac joint pain despite addressing all these factors. Unfortunately, attempts to use radio-frequency denervation procedures on the sacroiliac joint are fraught with difficulty because the segmental nerve supply is much larger than that for a facet joint, and so far has not proved to be effective. In the UK, currently there is no solution for this particular problem other than pain management. In some countries other than the UK, where hypermobility or instability has been clearly demonstrated, attempts have been made to fuse the joint, with varying degrees of success.

my experience

I am a 23-year-old female squash player, and although I work a ten-hour day in the City in an IT department, I consider myself to be very fit. However, I had been getting increasing pain down my left thigh to my knee, eased by playing squash and running around, only to get worse a few hours later. It was most painful when commuting by train into London because I often had to stand. I went to see a sports therapist at the squash club initially, who thought I had a muscle strain. When my left knee started to give way, I went to see my GP who found that I had slight wasting of the quadriceps and loss of the knee jerk on the affected side. He referred me to the musculoskeletal specialist privately at my request since I was insured, and requested early diagnosis and treatment. He diagnosed a probable disc prolapse with nerve root irritation at the third lumbar level (L3/4) and gave me a caudal epidural steroid injection. I was a lot better for a month but the pain gradually returned.

When I consulted the musculoskeletal doctor a second time, he ordered an MRI scan which confirmed the presence of a third and fourth lumbar level (L3/4) disc prolapse with an extruded fragment compressing the fourth lumbar (L4) root. He treated me with a nerve root block under X-ray control with a targeted dose of local anaesthetic mixed with steroid. Following this, I had excellent relief from pain and had no recurrence within a month. He advised me to keep my squash playing down to a minimum over the following months and to avoid any movements of the back towards extension. I found sitting to be no problem. Six weeks later, I was reviewed and was very happy with my progress and the specialist told me that the piece of disc material that was compressing the nerve was gradually disappearing as part of the natural healing process.

CHAPTER

7

Surgery and pain management

Is surgery appropriate?

In this book, we have explained that surgery is rarely indicated for most forms of back pain. The most commonly performed surgical operation is discectomy (see below) for disc prolapse (herniation), but surgery for disc prolapse is rarely essential. It is simply an option to be considered seriously when non-surgical treatment has not worked. Since the natural history for disc prolapse is gradual resolution over six months to one year, with or without surgery, one could avoid surgery altogether by 'sitting it out'. However, when nerve root pain is severe and not well controlled by epidural steroids or nerve root blocks, and the sufferer is unable to work or go about their normal activities for several weeks or months, the prospect of relief from going 'under the knife' becomes much more attractive. If there is a large central disc prolapse compressing the nerves controlling bladder and bowel function (cauda equina syndrome), there is no doubt that urgent surgical decompression is required. Fortunately, these situations are few and far between and for most people it is a difficult decision to weigh up the balance between whether they can tolerate the pain in anticipation of gradual recovery, or go for surgery.

myth
If you have weakness of muscles due to nerve root damage, this is more likely to recover if you have surgery.

fact
This is probably only true if surgery is done in the first 12 hours of nerve root compression. Following that, the damage is done and natural recovery occurs whether or not there is surgical decompression. In some instances, full recovery of muscle function does not occur. If the disc herniation is enlarging and there is progressive loss of nerve and therefore muscle function, surgical decompression should be considered early, but this situation is not commonly encountered.

myth
Having surgery will fix my back for good.

fact
All back surgeons should explain to you that disc surgery is done for relief of the pain in your leg due to the trapped nerve. They will not promise any relief of your back pain. This is because the pain in the back may be due to other mechanical factors which will not be addressed by simply removing the piece of prolapsed disc which is protruding into the spinal canal. If your pain is predominantly in the back, then this may mean that success from surgery will be less likely.

myth
If I go for surgery now, this will give me a better back in the future.

fact
In studies carried out comparing patients who opt for surgery versus non-surgical treatment, at one year there is only a slight difference in levels of pain and function. This difference diminishes, until by four years there is no difference between those who have had surgery and those who have not in terms of outcome.

myth
Back surgery is dangerous.

fact
Serious complications from disc surgery for the back are extremely rare (less than 1 in a 1000). There are, of course, the common complications of any general anaesthetic which may include wound infection, deep vein thrombosis, urinary retention or chest infection. However, the actual risks of back surgery are very low in terms of damage to the spine, spinal cord or nerves. The success rate in terms of relief of leg pain, which is usually almost instant, is something in the order of 85–90 per cent. Approximately 10 per cent do not seem to benefit, possibly because the nerve root has been too severely damaged or the mechanical back pain is a more significant factor. A small percentage – less than 5 per cent – develop scarring around the nerve root as a result of surgery and this may produce long-term activity-related pain in the back or leg due to tethering of the nerve root. This last problem is one of the more difficult situations to resolve. The degree of scarring is rarely much to do with the surgical technique; people vary enormously in their reaction to the mechanical stimulation of nerve tissue and dural tissue and it is not uncommon for people to develop scar tissue in relation to chronic disc problems, even without surgery. Recent studies have shown that a degree of fibrosis or scarring may occur in up to 30 per cent of all patients following disc surgery. Those who develop post-operative nerve root pain do not necessarily show any greater degree of scarring.

Alternatives to disc surgery

With the amount of media attention given to new medical technology, patients frequently hear about new techniques which may avoid surgery. The most tried and tested of these minimally invasive alternatives to disc surgery is chemonucleolysis. Since the early 1980s this has been used for certain kinds of disc prolapse to good effect. The preparation, derived from papaya, is an enzyme called chymopapain, and is injected into the centre of the disc which has prolapsed on to the nerve root. The enzyme digests the contents of the centre of the disc, thereby decompressing the disc space. The effects are more gradual than surgery, taking up to six to eight weeks and may, in the long term, lead to a slightly reduced disc size. In the short term, people may get some back spasms, although this is less likely since the size of the dose has been reduced. Occasionally, allergy to the enzyme may occur, so it is very important to screen patients for this risk in advance. The results compare very favourably with microdiscectomy (see below), except there is a higher recurrence rate and up to 15 per cent may eventually go on to have disc surgery.

Other minimally invasive techniques include the use of laser technology and radio-frequency currents through a bipolar electrode to induce a plasma state which literally vaporizes the centre of the disc to decompress from within. This technique is called 'RF Coblation Nucleoplasty', and is promising for the less severe disc protrusions which have not ruptured through the containing ligaments at the back of the spine.

However, simple discectomy or microdiscectomy, which involves the use of a dissecting microscope and a very small incision over the affected level, remains the gold standard in the treatment of disc problems. Once the cut through the skin and muscle has healed and the stitches have been removed 10 days later, people are free to go about their daily work. With the microdiscectomy, the wound is so small patients often go home the day after surgery.

I am a 42-year-old engineer and I was recently involved in a project that required a lot of driving. At the same time, my family and I had to move house, and during this period I developed increasingly troublesome pain in the left buttock, back of the thigh and occasionally down to the calf. The pain was worse on sitting and driving, and noticeably worse on any bending and leaning over activities.

My GP prescribed me painkillers and anti-inflammatory medication and encouraged me to take more exercise. I was referred for physiotherapy where 'sciatica' was diagnosed. I was given traction and McKenzie exercises. Initially, this seemed to help but, after a few weeks, when I was still getting settled into my new house and moving a lot of furniture, I got a lot worse.

When I went to see my GP she referred me to the musculoskeletal service. The triage therapist arranged an MRI to check for a disc problem and referred me to the musculoskeletal specialist for a possible epidural steroid injection. This injection worked well for ten days but the pain then came back. The MRI scan showed a large focal protrusion on the left side at the lowest level disc, L5/S1. So I was seen by a surgeon who agreed that an operation was the next step. I had to reduce my travelling by car for the next month and then went in for my operation – a microdiscectomy. This resulted in dramatic relief of the pain in my leg and I was able to stop taking all the painkillers! I was discharged from hospital within two days and was back working in my office by the eleventh day. I was advised not to do any heavy work or vigorous sport for the next six to eight weeks, which I followed, and am very happy to say that I made a full recovery.

Surgical treatment

The key to success in performing surgery is the selection of the right patients. The specialist must ensure that the patient's expectations are realistic and psychosocial factors which may interfere with progress and recovery must be addressed. Most specialists should be able to recognize the clear-cut clinical picture of a disc prolapse with nerve root compression and, with the aid of MRI scanning, be able to correlate the images obtained with the clinical picture. If non-surgical measures have failed, and these would include a trial of physiotherapy, injection therapy and the passage of time, appropriate disc surgery can be strongly recommended.

Spinal decompression surgery

People with spinal stenosis syndromes, causing narrowing of the central or lateral canal around the nerve root, may benefit from decompression. This is more likely to affect an elderly back pain sufferer with degenerative changes causing narrowing of disc space and growth of osteophytes which encroach on the root canal spaces. With an ageing population, there is an increasing awareness of the problem of stenosis causing **neurogenic claudication.**

neurogenic claudication
Pain and abnormal sensations arising from the nerves that are squeezed in a narrow spinal canal.

With this condition, an elderly sufferer will find they can only walk short distances before pain down the legs and loss of balance and control causes them to seek a park bench for immediate relief. The condition is really quite disabling and, if imaging investigations show one or often two levels of stenosis, surgical decompression may offer the best solution. Some patients are too old or infirm to consider surgery, in which case epidural (injection) steroid administration can help patients for up to six months at a time. Failing injection technique, patients can either adapt by adopting an increasingly bowed posture and use a stick to get about and limit their outside activities, or agree to surgery. Surgery involves the removal of a small piece of bone from the ring of bone at each level of the spine which has narrowed. This allows circulation to return to the nerves. There are no serious complications from this surgery and outcomes are invariably good, at least in the short term. There is a risk from removing too much bone and destabilizing the segments. This is something that a spine surgeon would be well aware of and therefore specialists tend to adopt a fairly conservative stance with this sort of surgery.

Chronic mechanical back pain

Surgical treatment for chronic mechanical back pain is the most controversial. Traditionally, surgeons have sought to fuse the so-called unstable or degenerate segments, either using bone graft or screws. Nowadays there is a profusion of techniques involving either or both of these combinations and including synthetic ligament stabilization methods. Each spinal surgeon has their preferred method of fusion and there is little indication that any of the new technology works better than the more traditional bone-grafting technique called 'postero-lateral fusion'. There are very few controlled trials on spinal fusion but those that have been performed recently show a moderate benefit at best.

How can I avoid spinal fusion?

As a result of the uncertainty surrounding surgery for chronic mechanical back pain and the fact that most people are reluctant to undergo such a radical treatment, a variety of minimally invasive intradiscal techniques for mechanical back pain have developed.

The source of the pain has to be identified accurately, and this can be done through the use of local anaesthetic blocking of specific structures, either the disc or the facet joints in most cases. Discography is used to diagnose the relevant disc as a source of pain. Plate 17 shows three-level discography with posterior annular tears in the upper two levels. However, not all specialists are

Q **I have been told my spine is degenerating and nothing can be done. Is this true?**

A Some patients are told that there is degeneration or wear and tear in the spine and there is nothing that can be done. Unfortunately, patients may go away with the misconception that their spine is so bad that even advanced spinal surgery cannot salvage the problem. This of course makes them feel worse about their back and even more hopeless. What is really meant is that surgery is simply not appropriate for this sort of problem, but it does not rule out other sources of help such as rehabilitation.

convinced of the reliability of this method and prefer to judge by the appearance of the discs on an MRI scan.

IDET

A large number of patients have tried techniques such as IDET (Intradiscal Electrothermal Therapy) to desensitize and stiffen the annulus fibrosis of the disc. Evidence of the benefit of this technique is still inconclusive, although it appears to be relatively safe. Other techniques using radio-frequency currents and similar electrode or catheter placements in the back of the disc, which is the most commonly painful area, are also being tried and tested.

DISC prosthesis

Perhaps the biggest and most exciting advance since the early 1990s has been the development of various types of disc prosthesis with which a painful disc can be entirely replaced. These prostheses will restore the disc space to its normal height and allow for an almost normal range of flexibility. Trials are being conducted on the long-term safety and effectiveness of these procedures and, although there are many anecdotes of great success with this technique, the jury is still out in terms of the long-term outcomes.

Q I have been told surgery is not appropriate – what do I do?

A If you have chronic back pain or leg pain and you have seen a surgical specialist who has told you quite definitely that he or she is not prepared to operate, it is very important to understand the reasons why. In the vast majority of cases, it is because the surgeon feels that there is nothing he or she can do that will offer any chance of success. If honest, he or she may admit that they cannot work out the cause for your continuing pain.

Furthermore, it has been shown time and time again that any form of spinal surgery should be done only with very clear indications, and only on patients who have a relatively normal psychosocial profile. It is quite common for good units to use various questionnaires and scales to determine whether a prospective candidate for surgery has a relatively normal or average psychometric profile. If a person is depressed, shows signs of abnormal illness or pain behaviour, excessive fear avoidance, is involved in litigation, receiving workers' compensation or fallen into the state benefits trap and is poorly motivated to recover, then the surgeon will be less keen to operate.

Stabilization procedures

The various forms of stabilization have been mentioned in reference to chronic mechanical back pain (see page 127). Although controversial, spinal stabilization techniques are essential in certain types of fracture and tumour management. Furthermore, unstable segments which are slipping forwards (spondylolisthesis) require stabilization to avoid damage to the spinal cord or nerves. There is a vast amount of research and clinical experience with spine stabilization techniques in these indications and there is no doubt about their value.

Vertebroplasty and balloon kyphoplasty

These techniques of injection of bone cement into the vertebral body are used for compression fractures resulting from osteoporosis which are not healing and are still painful. Vertebroplasty simply involves the injection of bone cement through the fracture line into the vertebral body under X-ray control. This appears to relieve the pain very quickly although care has to be taken that the cement does not leak out of the bone into other areas where it may cause complications. Balloon kyphoplasty involves the insertion of a balloon into the vertebral body, and pumping this up with cement to actually reduce the deformity of the wedge compression. These techniques are promising for persistently painful osteoporotic compression fractures, although their exact place in clinical management remains to be defined since the vast majority of patients with osteoporotic compression fracture make a full recovery within four to six weeks of onset, albeit with some loss of upright posture due to the wedging of the vertebra.

my experience

As a 53-year-old woman, I had suffered low back pain for many years. I worked as a care assistant in a nursing home, and my own family was fully grown. I had increasing periods of time off work over the preceding two years due to my back pain. A particularly severe episode after lifting a heavy patient resulted in pain shooting down the outer aspect of my right leg. This did not respond to any of the previous therapy that I had relied on. This included manual therapy, exercises, acupuncture and injection therapy, although all of these had produced some temporary relief.

I was referred to a local neurosurgeon who performed all the spinal surgery in my district. He took MRI scans, identified a moderately severe disc degeneration at both lower lumbar levels, L4/5 and L5/S1, with marked narrowing and a diffuse disc bulge at L4/5 which was more marked on the right, the L5 root clearly being irritated. He decided to operate and remove the bulging disc material at L4/5 and at the same time to decompress the L5 root canal by undercutting the L5/S1 facet joint.

Unfortunately I only experienced relief of pain in my leg for six weeks until it started to return. Since the operation I have had a lot of low back pain, perhaps worse than before, and now the leg pain has become even worse within ten weeks of surgery. The pain in my leg was related mainly to any increased activity such as walking. The neurosurgeon tried an epidural and a nerve root block to no avail. He arranged a second MRI scan which showed considerable scarring in the spinal canal at L4/5 and L5/S1. He said there was no more he could do and referred me to the pain clinic.

Chronic pain syndrome

Surgery is not always a viable option and perhaps one of the most common reasons for surgery not being offered is that an acute pain has become chronic and this has led to sensitization or 'wind-up' of the central nervous system. In simple terms, this means that the pain is no longer coming from actual tissue damage as in a bruise, cut or burn but is originating within the nervous system itself. This is a complex process that is difficult to understand, even for doctors. It is described in as simple a way as possible below. Figure 7.1 shows a model that was developed in the 1960s by Melzack and Wall to demonstrate pain pathways from the periphery to the brain. It is called the pain gate theory. For reasons not yet fully understood, the normal balance of control operating at the spinal level becomes disturbed. The descending or **inhibitory** messages from the brain are less effective. The touch and pressure sensations from the skin and muscles no longer work to reduce the pain 'traffic' passing through the gate (boxed area) in the **dorsal horn** of the spinal cord. This is the result of changes in certain chemicals and in the development of new connections. Consequently, the volume of pain messages ascending the spine to the brain increases, that is to say their onward passage is **facilitated**.

With chronic pain syndrome there is an increased pain network which is picking up signals from the periphery, i.e. skin, joint or muscle, which is not necessarily to do with pain or the threat of harm. Movement, stretch, compression and light touch all send messages to the brain, but in abnormal pain processing any or all of these signals may be misinterpreted as painful. This effect appears to be initiated at the dorsal horn level in the spinal cord but soon has effects which can be seen or detected at a more central level in the brain – that is

dorsal horn

The dorsal horn is the area of the spinal cord where sensory input from the periphery relays with other nerves, some of which descend from the brain. It is the location of the 'pain gate mechanism'.

inhibitory and facilitatory pathways

Nerve tracts in the spinal cord that may either suppress or encourage the summation of pain impulses.

disturbed sleep and increased anxiety, and the pain centres in the brain appear to be switched on and overactive. A specialist will be able to detect these changes by finding increased sensitivity of the skin or subcutaneous tissues on palpation. Normal movements unrelated to the original problem all provoke pain. Circulation to the skin may change, causing temperature and colour changes, as well as abnormal sweating or dry skin. The quality of the pain described by the patient changes from simple terms such as sharp and dull to burning, tearing, drawing, gnawing and such like. Sometimes light touch or even the pressure of clothing or bed clothes sets off severe pain and spasms.

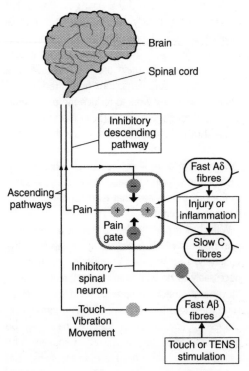

| **Figure 7.1** Pain gate theory (Melzack and Wall).

Perhaps the best-known example of a chronic pain disorder is phantom limb pain, when an amputee still experiences pain from the leg which has long since gone. In order to remove the leg originally, some main nerves had to be cut, and sometimes abnormal growth occurs at the cut ends in the stump and neuromas (tumours on a nerve cell sheath) form which become hypersensitive and signal pain messages at random into the system. This example, where nerve damage itself may cause a chronic pain syndrome, is called '**neuropathic pain**' which is distinct from '**nociceptive pain**' where there is ongoing tissue damage or injury.

There are various forms of chronic pain but possibly the most common is neuropathic pain caused by actual nerve damage. This may occur in conditions such as diabetes and shingles where the nerve cells or nerve fibres are directly attacked. However, in other back conditions, chronic pain syndromes develop which are not clearly due to nerve damage and there may be no actual signs of nerve damage. If this is found in an upper or lower limb, i.e. an extremity, it would be called 'complex regional pain syndrome' (CRPS). When applied to the spine, which is non-extremity, it may be referred to as CRPS Type Three.

The key points of CRPS Type Three are:

1 Surgery is not appropriate
2 A chronic pain disorder has developed
3 Psychosocial factors are interfering with function and the chances of success with any single intervention or procedure.

This kind of problem needs to be dealt with by an experienced clinician with some knowledge of pain management principles – the pain specialist.

neuropathic pain
Pain that arises from damaged or abnormally functioning nerve tissue.

nociceptive pain
Pain that arises from stimulation of a pain receptor by an unpleasant event, e.g. a cut, burn, bruise or pinch.

Q My specialist says I have a chronic pain syndrome. Can the misbehaving nerves be switched off?

A If only it were that simple. Unfortunately structural changes will have occurred in the organization of the pain pathways and they take a long time to normalize and, in some cases, never do completely.

fact
Most people who have a normally functioning nervous system have very much the same physical thresholds for nociceptive stimulation. However, research has recently shown that there is a genetic factor which codes for certain enzymes in the nervous system and which can alter tolerance of pain. Therefore, some patients will have a lower tolerance of chronic pain than others. Perhaps this is not surprising since there clearly are differences between individuals in their ability to endure pain.

Pain services

Referral to the pain service is appropriate for back pain sufferers with moderate to severe pain levels, which has become chronic. It is for those who have failed to respond to simple therapies and interventions, in whom surgery has been ruled out as not necessary or appropriate, or which has already been tried and failed. It is probably most appropriate for those who are unable to live with the problem, not coping, and becoming increasingly disabled by it.

Most larger district or general hospitals around the UK now have a pain service. Ideally, a comprehensive pain service will include the following professionals:

◇ A pain specialist, usually with background training in anaesthetics and the specialty of management of acute and chronic pain
◇ A nurse specialist
◇ A physiotherapy specialist
◇ A clinical psychologist
◇ Sometimes a member of the musculoskeletal services.

Patients should be assessed by a multi-professional team to assess their suitability for either further investigation or a form of pain management. Pain management can be offered in a variety of different ways:

1 An outpatient programme incorporating psychological principles of pain management and activation to return to full function
2 An inpatient programme with residential accommodation
3 Pain intervention may be considered by the pain clinic; it may be some form of interventional procedure such as nerve root block or radio-frequency facet denervation.

my experience

I am a 65-year-old retired toolmaker, and I have suffered increasing low back pain over the last ten or fifteen years. These episodes usually cleared with exercises and manipulation but over the last year or two, the pain had become constant. In particular, it was aggravated by playing golf, which was the one recreation I had been looking forward to on retirement. I was taking increasing amounts of pain medication and generally felt rather despondent.

I went to see my GP who examined me and found evidence of a very stiff back with tight lumbar extensor muscles and with tenderness over the paravertebral tissues and deeper joint structures in the lower lumbar region. There were no signs of any nerve root tension and he said that I could bend very well for my age, without pain. Since I had not benefited from any of the physical therapies I had tried in the preceding year, my GP decided to refer me straight to the pain clinic. There, I was seen by the pain specialist who noted the physical findings and looked at my previous X-rays which showed general wear and tear in the lower lumbar spine. He offered me a diagnostic test which was to inject the facet joints with a small dose of local anaesthetic and steroid under X-ray control. This was successful in relieving my pain for nearly two months by which time it started to recur.

> The pain specialist recommended a specific exercise programme to help unload the facet joints in the lower lumbar region by reducing the lordosis, or hollowness, in the lower back both in standing and walking as well as through flexion exercises. This again helped me for a while but the pain seemed to return in the long run and I still could not play golf properly.
>
> The specialist then decided to perform a further diagnostic test using a small dose of local anaesthetic delivered to the target nerve that carried pain messages from the facet joints. This seemed to abolish the pain completely for the duration of the anaesthetic. The pain specialist was satisfied that this would indicate a good chance of response to radio-frequency facet denervation. This treatment was arranged on the next available date and I went in for a small day case procedure in the local hospital. Within a month of the procedure, I felt I could move and walk more freely, and furthermore I had played my first round of golf without provoking back pain! I have continued to do my exercises and have remained free of pain to this day.

An inpatient programme is a more comprehensive programme offered at only a few centres and which may last between two to four weeks. The patient will be admitted to the unit with a group of other fellow sufferers and will be encouraged to take part in the group activities throughout the day. Being removed from the normal environment at home and being given support and encouragement from an expert team, as well as sharing problems with fellow sufferers, may give an enormous boost to motivation and hope.

functional rehabilitation
An approach that focuses on function, rather than pain or damage, to return people to a more normal life.

Simpler forms of pain management are called **'functional rehabilitation'** programmes, and can be suitable for people who are less severely disabled but need a combination of psychological management, education and physical rehabilitation.

What else may I expect from the pain service?

The pain specialist will be able to advise on medication. Unfortunately, many patients slide from acute back pain to chronic back pain, relying on much the same kind of pain medications that are more appropriate for acute pain. (Acute back pain is classified as that which is within 12 weeks of onset and chronic back pain is that which continues for more than 12 weeks.) Traditionally, pain medications based on codeine or opiates have been discouraged for chronic back pain because of the risk of side effects or physical and psychological dependency.

However, for severe chronic pain, there is clearly a trade-off between the debilitating effects of coping with chronic uncontrolled, severe pain and the possible side effects from strong analgesics such as morphine-type drugs. The pain specialist will attend to a number of important factors to help the sufferer regain a feeling of control over their life.

Sleep disturbance

Sleep disturbance due to pain or other factors reduces quality of life considerably. The use of low-dose tricyclics such as amitriptyline (normally used as an antidepressant in higher doses) can have significant benefit. It may serve to reduce nerve sensitivity as well as relaxing muscles and having some sedative effect at night. It is often given in a low dosage.

Explore your thoughts, beliefs and attitudes

People who develop chronic pain from whatever source may lose hope and motivation and develop a negative thinking pattern. They may also have certain unhelpful concepts about the meaning of pain – that hurt means harm, that all pain is to be avoided, and a variety of other beliefs that may obstruct progress. The specialist will need to explore the patient's understanding of their present problem and deal with the various confused messages that may have been given from different practitioners. The most important aspects of an initial consultation are for the specialist to listen to the story and take time to dispel misconceptions, increase understanding about the nature of chronic pain, and agree on common goals. In other words, the patient becomes part of the team in this process and the doctor becomes their advocate.

---

myth
The doctor thinks it's all in my mind.

fact
Some patients may get the idea that as soon as the specialist talks in terms of psychological approaches to manage chronic pain that this is a humiliating slur on their honesty and integrity, that the pain is not real or is not physical in nature. Nothing could be further from the truth. In one sense, from a scientific point of view, all kinds of pain are 'all in the mind' because pain is an experience of the nervous system which is processed and interpreted and reaches consciousness through activities of your brain. In another sense, all pain is entirely in the body because your nervous system is integrated as a network in almost all the tissues throughout your body. Therefore, pain is a mind/body experience. Much research has shown how the application of mental techniques can influence the pain experience, especially if physical approaches have failed. For example, it has recently been shown that simply focusing on a physical pain tends to enhance its magnitude and dominance in your consciousness. The pain centres in the brain light up when you give your pain more attention. This can be toned down by distracting yourself from the pain, attaching less importance to it, and getting on with other things. This active process starts to reduce the activity of the pain centres. In other words, it is possible to turn the 'volume' down.

Q Is there some sort of injection or surgery to the nerves that can fix my problem?

A Before embarking on any such efforts it is important to understand that there is no 'fix' to your problem, only strategies to help you gain better control of the pain experience and reduce its effect on your life.

A pain intervention

If there is a continuing source of nociceptive pain, some interventional procedures may be used additionally to settle certain acute aspects of the whole pain syndrome. Such pain intervention is only likely to be used in the absence of neuropathic pain and a relatively normal psychosocial profile.

Self-help techniques

The use of a TENS (transcutaneous electrical nerve stimulation) or similar device often helps people with chronic pain become less dependent on medication. It is a relatively cheap and effective form of self-help which requires some training for the patient to use effectively. In one study of its application in a pain service, up to 50 per cent of patients obtained some relief from the use of a TENS machine. However, it is difficult to predict what kind of pain syndromes or particular kind of TENS application works best. Surface electrodes applied at the maximum sites of pain pass a small electrical signal through the skin and tissues which may serve to block the 'pain gate' as shown in the Melzack and Wall model of 1964 (see Figure 7.1).

Other self-help techniques include relaxation, visual imagery and setting of achievable targets on a day-to-day basis.

Patients selected for pain management programmes tend to be those who are not coping with their present level of pain and the resultant disability. The main aim of these programmes is to learn to live with the problem without the expectation of a magic fix or cure. If a patient is still preoccupied with the possibility of a cure they may not be ready to learn about accepting the problem and beginning the process of maximizing quality of life and physical function. It is emphasized that these programmes do not aim to reduce the pain intensity but to enhance the quality of life and physical and social functioning. They will help patients emerge from the downward spiral of inactivity, depression and despair through to gradual re-adjustment to a new form of life.

Mary, the 53-year-old care assistant with chronic low back pain, has now been off work for just over six months (see page 130). The back surgery had failed, and the neurosurgeon had said that the scarring at the site of operation was probably the cause of her continuing problems. She had her first appointment with the pain specialist. The specialist listened to Mary's account of 20 years of increasing relapses of back pain and difficulties in coping at work and home.

Mary's family circumstances included a husband who had retired early for medical reasons with a bad back, a 29-year-old son who was living at home, and a mother-in-law whom she had to look after on a daily basis. Mary had now become quite depressed and was taking quite a lot of dihydrocodeine tablets for the pain, and these had caused chronic constipation. She was not sleeping well and had become very inactive, taking rests during the day. She admitted to losing hope and didn't feel that her husband or son gave her very much support or understanding.

The pain specialist listened to Mary's story and showed her sympathy, giving her plenty of time and taking great care during the physical examination not to aggravate the pain too much. The specialist found much limitation of movement and stiffness in the back and hips. She noted that Mary was overweight and had quite a marked limitation of straight leg-raising on the left side, provoking the root pain. Mary also had widespread tenderness of the soft tissues around the lumbar and pelvic area. The pain specialist explained that she could not cure Mary's problem or necessarily get rid of the pain, but by taking a holistic approach to deal with all the factors, she believed that Mary was capable of a much better quality of life and function.

The specialist recommended an inpatient pain management programme. Mary's husband and son

my experience

would have to look after themselves and the mother-in-law for a month while Mary came in for full rehabilitation. The pain specialist explained that this was not a new treatment, but that Mary would have to take full responsibility for her involvement to get the most out of it. In the meantime, she started Mary on antidepressant medication (tricyclics) at a moderate dosage level to improve her sleep, help her depression and reduce the nerve pain. The specialist recommended cutting down the codeine and replacing this with tramadol.

After a month, the specialist started Mary on Pregabalin for neuropathic pain. About two months later Mary was able to attend the pain management programme and was already feeling more hopeful. She participated fully in the programme, which included psychological input emphasizing self-help techniques and a graduated programme of physical activity and exercises. By the time Mary left, she understood her condition much better. On review two months later, Mary was much brighter, talked less about her pain and more about what she was now able to do. She had already achieved three of the five goals that she had set with the physiotherapist as realistic targets for the first three months. She was walking 3 km each day, going to dance classes with her husband and had started an evening course in IT. She intended to go back to work in the care home in an administrative capacity. She rarely slept during the day and had lost weight. Most importantly, Mary now accepted that she was able to live with the current level of pain and was still able to look forward to a reasonable quality of life.

CHAPTER

8

Living with back pain

If you have tried all the different specialists and physical therapists, or even had surgery, and still have back or leg pain related to your back problem, you may have to face the reality of learning to live with the pain. For many people, this is extremely difficult, particularly if the pain is severe or disabling. If you are not coping, then some sort of pain management approach is worth seeking out. If you are coping, in the sense that you are able to lead a life of reasonable quality, maintain some of your usual activities and go to work, then you are adapting to the circumstances.

If you are not coping or you are perhaps still hoping that there is a cure for back pain out there, you may be tempted to try all the different offers of help advertised in the media or on the internet. You might spend many years and a lot more money before realizing that this is a fruitless search; on the other hand, you might get lucky. At some point, however, there comes a time when you may have to face the reality that, despite all the miracles of modern or complementary medicine, there is not a cure for every kind of back pain. This chapter is designed to help you to help yourself.

The important exception to this applies to those who have had some form of back surgery for the first time. If the operation has not solved your problem, you may wonder whether another operation or surgeon will succeed. This depends on the reason why your surgery did not work:

✧ The operation may have been inappropriate
✧ You may have been given unrealistic expectations (following simple disc surgery, 50 per cent of patients continue to have some back pain)
✧ There may have been a technical problem or error (wrong level of the spine, inadequate clearance, a bleed or dural leak of cerebrospinal fluid)
✧ You may have developed scarring which is usually unavoidable
✧ You may have developed an infection or had a recurrence of disc prolapse or new disc protrusion at a different level
✧ There may be nerve root damage or some unexplained reason for the pain not to settle following a technically successful operation (most often the case).

If you have had a discectomy or spinal decompression surgery which has not worked, it is important to enquire further with the back surgeon. Unfortunately, some spinal surgeons are reluctant to admit their failures or to initiate further investigations into those patients who are having ongoing problems. In this situation, we would advise you to take the results of your scans, obtain a summary of your operation, and seek a second opinion from a recommended spinal surgeon. It may be useful to do a further

MRI (Magnetic Resonance Imaging) scan with the addition of Gadolinium enhancement which helps to separate out the appearance of scarring from disc material. There may have been a period of relief followed by a relapse which suggests a further disc prolapse, either at the same level of the spine or, more commonly, at an adjacent level. When these important searches have been made and all other possible forms of help have been considered, the end result may be the same – you will have to be prepared to learn to live with the problem. At this stage, if the pain is still a significant problem, the spinal surgeon will probably refer you to a pain service for further help and advice.

Acceptance

The first step to learning to live with back pain is to accept your predicament as it is now. Acceptance means:

◇ Recognizing your current limitations and not dwelling on your past level of fitness as if you can turn back the clock
◇ Adjusting your lifestyle rather than constantly pushing yourself to the limits
◇ Taking responsibility for your back, getting to know what it likes and what it doesn't like, and getting to know the pain and negotiating with it as an ally rather than a foe. Ceasing the search for a cure and getting on with your life.

You may feel that you have become old, at least in your lifestyle, before your time. We all have to grow old and accept the increasing handicaps and restrictions some time, and we may as well learn to do it gracefully.

Some people have difficulty believing the pain is real and, therefore through this self-doubt, do not communicate clearly to friends, doctors and significant others. They may be denying the pain's reality or think that they are going mad – this is particularly likely to happen if the doctor or specialist doesn't understand the pain and doubts the sufferer's veracity. Others become very angry and refuse to accept the pain and constantly fight it which leads to problems of frustration with flare-ups (see below).

Stop blaming others

The second step to learning to live with back pain is to allow your current pain and disability to be integrated more fully into your social and family life. This means letting people know what you can and cannot do. As soon as you have more realistic expectations of your own capabilities, others will be able to learn your limitations. If you feel you have developed your back pain as the result of some injury or accident through no fault of your own, you may be harbouring some feelings of blame or bitterness against a third party. In order to live with your problem you must learn to forgive and forget. This is particularly difficult for those people who are still involved in litigation or some sort of injury compensation; so the sooner this is settled, the better.

Clear communication

Communicating your pain and disability is important and can have a variety of effects. It is important not to be too stoical when consulting your doctor or he may never be able to understand the true impact on your life. Being miserable and going on about it all the time may drive him or her, and others, away.

'Killing' with kindness

You may sometimes get more attention than is actually good for you. Research has shown that in couple relationships where one partner has a chronic pain problem, if the other partner is over-attentive or too solicitous to their every need, it will actually have a counterproductive effect. You may get too dependent on him or her and be less able to help yourself.

The snag of diagnosis

Another aspect that many people find difficult is the lack of a clear diagnosis. Some back pains are insoluble and, despite the best efforts of back pain experts, a clear-cut source or cause cannot be found. On your journey with back pain you may have encountered some health care professionals who have doubted your honesty or integrity, or who seemed not to believe the extent of your problem. The best way forward is to agree on a dignified explanation of your back pain with a trusted doctor – one that is acceptable to you both. Call the explanation whatever is preferred; accept the label and it will get you 'off the hook'. The hook is still believing you have to prove you have an identifiable problem at every new encounter with a doctor or health care professional. As one physician asked, 'How can you get better if you are still trying to prove that you are ill?' This particularly refers to people with controversial conditions like fibromyalgia and chronic fatigue syndrome, but it can equally apply to chronic back pain.

Pace yourself

The third step to learning to live with back pain is to learn to pace yourself. Most pain management programmes will incorporate education on this strategy. Simply put, this means that you are able to avoid the peaks and troughs of the pain by regulating the amount of activity that you do over the day. Most people have good days and bad days. It is tempting to try and fit all those jobs you can't do on the bad days into a good day, inevitably overloading yourself and getting a flare-up. In a flare-up, you rest and lose fitness and a sense of control over the pain. You are likely to develop negative thoughts, of which you should become aware early on in order to nip them in the bud. It helps to see a flare-up as part of the problem, and to learn to plan for this event by having extra rescue medication available, anticipating these setbacks and seeing them as part of the condition.

> **Q** **I can't tell what causes a flare-up so how can I avoid it?**
>
> **A** You can't always avoid flare-ups – they are part of a chronic pain disorder, as are good days and bad days. However, keeping a pain diary of your activities and pain levels for a month may help you to recognize some of the triggers, especially when the flare-up follows a day or two later rather than instantly. Through careful monitoring you should be able to identify the level of activity and exercise that you can tolerate before the pain worsens.

Coping with flare-ups

Inevitably flare-ups will occur, and it is your attitude to them that counts. Everyday demands such as visitors, shopping, cleaning, family visits and access to shops and supermarkets may all affect just how much you can regulate your activities on a daily level in order to reduce the risk of a flare-up.

In the event of a flare-up try not to just 'down tools' and walk off in disgust, but maintain a modicum of exercise or you will lose fitness. This may involve periods of mild or moderate activity with short periods of rest. Consider a massage or similar soothing therapy. Instead of punishing yourself for getting it wrong, pamper yourself a little. Use the '**downtime**' to practise that new relaxation sequence or work a little more on improving your posture.

downtime
Refers to time spent flat on your back resting during the day.

Obstacles to pacing

pacing
A strategy for maintaining a steady level of activity without the peaks and troughs that risk causing flare-ups of pain.

When trying to **pace** yourself, your basic beliefs can get in the way. A common scenario is when you start a job in the garden which you feel you must finish – 'A job worth doing is worth doing well'. As a result, you spend an extra two hours working and overloading your back. If you exceed your limits, you will pay the price with back pain aggravation. Unfortunately, aggravations may last two or three days or sometimes longer, and so it is possible to fall back into a slough of despondency.

Another common belief is, 'If I start something I must finish it'. Why not break up complex and demanding jobs such as hoovering the living room into parts? Hoover one half, have a break, and them come back to finish the other half later. Perfectionists tend to pay dearly for their admirable qualities, but perfection is rarely achievable, so lower your sights and have fewer flare-ups. Flare-ups lead to negative thinking about the condition and to a loss of hope. Chronic back pain, in particular, is prone to erratic and often unpredictable fluctuations. This may make it difficult to plan the day or week ahead. Therefore, part of the pacing strategy is to make allowances for these unpredictable fluctuations.

Prioritize

Make a list of the things you plan to do, and then strike out all the items on the bottom half of the list. Through prioritization and setting limits like this, you will give yourself a little extra reserve which you may need if your back is playing up more than usual.

Goal-setting

The fourth step to learning to live with back pain involves setting goals. If you are optimistic, and ambitious, you may tend to set your goals too high. On the other hand, if you are feeling helpless and hopeless, you may not have any goals at all. It is important to spend time each week reflecting on the little goals that are achievable. Choose things you really want to do, not just 'ought-to's'. These may range from doing the small DIY job in your home through taking a half-hour drive to see a friend or relative to, even better for your circulation, a half-hour walk to the shop and back.

Achieving these little goals will give you a feeling of accomplishment and greater confidence. Perhaps next week you might be able to set your targets a little higher, but be careful not to overdo it. It is important to share your goals with friends and your doctor or carer. By making other people aware of what you are trying to achieve and agreeing with your partner how to achieve your goal, you will increase the chance of getting there. It is useful to have a small list of short-term goals, and then to work on a list of medium-term goals such as those you might achieve in the next few months. Some people find it helpful to put this in the context of longer-term goals over the next year or two, or even over the next five years. However, the most important thing is to find the right

Q My doctor says I must become independent. But when I get a flare-up I really need help. How am I supposed to manage?

A Your doctor is expressing a general principle which cannot apply to everyone or even anyone all of the time. Don't be proud; when you need help, ask for it. It is not a sign of weakness, and people usually like to help out.

Q How can I ever achieve my goals with this back pain getting in the way?

A A thousand-mile journey begins with the first step – break down your goals into bite-sized chunks.

balance from day to day. You may feel you have failed today, but tomorrow is a new day and you can adjust your current goals according to your experience – keep trying.

Focusing

fact
People often travel to opposite corners of the globe to avoid their problems, only to find it doesn't work. They are still the same person. Your pain is a backdrop to your present life, colouring your experience, but it isn't you. Don't let the problem distract you from focusing on the other important areas in your life that need attention.

Do not focus on your pain. This is the fifth step to learning to live with back pain. Try to find hobbies or interests that are totally absorbing; anything that serves to distract from the pain will be very effective. For some people, focusing on the pain has become a habit developed over many months or years. You will realize that this serves no useful purpose since the pain will be there anyway, either in the foreground or in the background.

You will already have learned that trying to lead a normal life and engage in normal activities will not injure or damage the structure of your back, and so dwelling on the pain and its implications is simply a waste of time. Chronic pain can tend to make a sufferer rather self-centred and sometimes socially isolated; it is important to get out and become aware of other people's situations. Very often it is surprising how many other people are managing with painful situations in their lives. Spending a little time helping them, or listening to their troubles, can be a welcome distraction from your own problems. Many people who have given up work due to chronic pain problems enjoy doing voluntary work in a hospice, hospital or workshop setting, deriving great satisfaction from helping others. There is always someone worse off than yourself.

Pain medication

The sixth step to learning to live with back pain is to take your pain medication regularly. If you are experiencing pain which is difficult to tolerate for most of the day, it is important to take your pain medication on a time-contingent basis. Do not use painkillers as a patch or remedy for a flare-up of pain. Instead, take your medication at regular intervals throughout the day, even if the pain has not broken through to an intolerable level before the next dose. This will help you to keep control of the use of medication and to maintain better control of the overall level of pain over the 24-hour period. If the pain makes you restless and agitated, such that you cannot concentrate properly, then you may need to seek further advice on improving pain control through medication.

For neuropathic pain, there are two relatively new medications available on the market – gabapentin and pregabalin. Either of these can calm down the nerve membrane excitability to a point where the worst aspects of pain can be ameliorated.

Do not expect to get 100 per cent relief of pain from any medication. At best, standard pain medications will relieve the pain by about half. Try to be content with the relative relief such medication gives. If you are receiving strong pain medication which is giving you side effects, consult your doctor for advice about adjusting dosage or type of drug. Obtaining adequate pain relief and avoiding side effects can be a delicate balance, but your doctor or pain specialist should be able to help with this.

Simple self-help remedies

As the last step in learning to live with back pain, self-help remedies can be very effective. Many of these have been discussed in the earlier chapters for the treatment of the acute onset of back pain. However, they may be just as useful for long-term pain.

Heat-packs

A heat-pack applied to the affected area may relieve muscle spasm. Wheat bags, the type that can be warmed up quickly in the microwave, may be the best way of obtaining a ready-made heat-pack. Hot water bottles, unfortunately, are all too prone to cause skin burns and may occasionally leak.

Relaxation and massage

Relaxation and massage are important ways of calming and centering yourself. If you have never learned to relax physically and mentally, ask your doctor for a recommendation to an appropriate therapist, or attend a course in relaxation for living which is offered through many community centres. Relaxation massage, aromatherapy and other gentle so-called holistic therapies can serve to calm the system on a temporary basis.

Sleep

'Sleep is the only medicine,' Socrates said in the fifth century BC. It is important to make sure that you are getting enough sleep, and to try to avoid resting and sleeping for long periods in the day which will make it more difficult to sleep at night and will encourage bad habits. Your doctor may be able to help with the right kind of medication to improve the quality of sleep. Obtaining four or five hours of deep, relaxed sleep is enormously restorative.

> **myth**
> When I am tired I should lie down and rest.

> **fact**
> Tiredness is due to many factors – some emotional such as depressed feelings, and some physiological such as the strain of coping with chronic pain. Other causes include lack of fitness and poor quality sleep. Tiredness needs analysing carefully before you simply give in to it.

Exercise

Traditionally, the benefits of exercise have been severely underrated for chronic musculoskeletal pain. Exercise is now recognized as one of the essential ingredients of pain management. Maintaining a modicum of strength, flexibility and cardiovascular fitness are perhaps the most vital results of exercise. If you have not had the benefit of a rehabilitation programme, you may find some help from a fitness instructor in a local gym, or the local physiotherapy department may run an outpatient rehabilitation programme to which your doctor could refer you. This would help to develop an exercise programme customized to your own needs and limitations from which you can build up small goals of achievement.

Find your baseline levels

The key principle for exercise is to start at the **baseline level** of activity – that which does not worsen the pain either immediately or a day or two later. For example, if weak leg muscles have been identified as a target to focus on, you might start with five half-depth knee bends. If this is well tolerated three days later, you might try seven or ten until you reach a point just below the level at

baseline levels
The level of activity or exercise that you can manage most days without increasing your pain intensity.

Q **Exercise makes my pain worse. Why should I do it?**

A You probably haven't been advised correctly about how to start exercising gently. Alternatively, there may be a little adjustment period (up to three months) during which some of the tissues will react to normal stretch because they have become stiff and inflexible.

which an aggravation is triggered. If seven is the baseline, this is incorporated into the exercise routine which may initially be done only two to three times a week. With repeated practice, fitness and strength improve, and gradually the frequency (times per week) or the intensity (number of repetitions) is increased. It may take three months to notice a difference in functioning, so do not give up too soon.

Baseline levels need to be found for walking, cooking and shopping, as well as for specific exercises. For more complex exercise such as golf, baseline levels for each component are obtained – try so many swings of the club in a session, play a limited number of holes and see how many holes can be walked or covered with a buggy or trolley. Often it can be the stopping to place the tee or pick the ball out of the hole that cause setbacks until these actions can be done correctly. In other words, technique of exercise has to be attended to as well as duration, intensity and frequency. Rest assured that the benefits far outweigh the risks – with a little perseverance and good advice, greater well-being, enhanced mood and tolerance of daily activities will be achieved through the production of endorphins (the body's own natural painkiller), metabolism of stress hormones, and efficient muscles.

Posture

Most people do not sit or stand in good postures, but with chronic pain it is easy to get into bad habits. Sitting on one buttock to lean away from the side of pain may reduce pain in the short term, but it soon leads to tension and strain higher up the spine. Likewise, standing on one leg to reduce weight bearing on the painful side is only a short-term solution. In the long term it creates problems that can escalate.

Trying to correct postural bad habits may not be easy in the first instance. Soft tissues adapt to sustained static strain by shortening and tightening and so it may hurt when you start straightening these areas out. Here are some basic points to follow:

1 Imagine a line of string attached to the crown of your head. Let it draw you upwards towards the ceiling, just forward from the vertical. Allow the neck and trunk to follow naturally.
2 Release the upper neck to allow a small nodding movement of the head.
3 Bring your chest forward so that your whole trunk aligns under head and neck.
4 Release the pelvis by rotating gently backwards if standing, or forwards if sitting, until it is in line with your spine (the direction and degree of movement will vary according to your habitual posture).
5 If standing, unlock the knees a fraction so that they remain slightly bent. Your weight should be coming through the balls of your feet.
6 Finally shrug your shoulders up, and lower them downwards and outwards, so they hang freely like the arms of a jacket hung by its loop on a peg.

Practise these steps regularly throughout the day, and the new posture will begin to feel more natural. The key is to use the visual image of the line of string to draw you upwards effortlessly, and to find the mid-range position of pelvis.

Specific exercises

Standing – half-depth knee bends
With feet slightly wider apart than your hips, keeping a straight back, bend at the knees about halfway to a full squat position and straighten again. Repeat ten times.

Deep breathing

Bring your arms out wide and upwards above your head while breathing in slowly and deeply. Make sure your belly moves out as you breathe in, indicating a full downward movement of your diaphragm before your chest inflates. Breathe out as you bring your arms down along the same path. Repeat ten times.

Rollover trunk flexion

From a full upright position, bend your head followed by your neck, upper back, mid-back and lower back, consciously releasing your back muscles in a slow fluent movement until you are hanging over in a fully bent position. Now straighten slowly from the base of your spine, bringing your pelvis under your spine through the action of your abdominals, uncurling your spine in reverse sequence. Repeat ten times.

Rotation of trunk

With legs firmly placed either side of the seat of your chair to lock your pelvis, straighten your spine fully, fold your arms and rotate your trunk slowly as far as you can one way as you breathe out. Breathe in on return and then rotate the other way. Rotate each way five times.

Rocking the pelvis forward and back

Sitting upright on a chair with your feet flat on the floor, roll slowly back on your sitting bones and then forward as far as you can. Now find the mid-position and familiarize yourself with this.

Lying with knees bent, gently flatten the small of your back to the floor and hold for ten seconds. Repeat ten times.

Walking an extra 50 m on alternate days, spending an extra five minutes on some gentle yoga stretches, or doing an extra ten repetitions of half-depth knee bends from week to week will accumulate to quite significant gains in strength, fitness and flexibility over a period of six months to one year. Learn to be flexible with your exercise programme to avoid flare-ups – pace yourself.

Relaxation sequence

This can be done either sitting or lying flat, whichever is most comfortable. Find a quiet place and time when you will not be disturbed. Check out your body, scanning for areas of tension or discomfort, and make any final adjustments of posture and clothing. Close your eyes and become aware of your breathing, the slow rise and fall of your belly as you breathe in and out. Notice any sounds around you – observe them and let any thoughts about them and any other intruding thoughts pass through your mind and dissipate with each **out breath**.

Starting with your feet, focus on how they feel, any areas of tension and, as you breathe out, let the tension go. Repeat this process with your legs, knees, thighs and hips, allowing plenty of time for each out breath to let go of the tension and discomfort.

Move on to the pelvis, lower abdomen, upper abdomen, chest and neck. Now move to the face and scalp, the mouth, tongue and eyes, until you have been through every area of your body.

Now you are feeling heavy and loose, warm and relaxed, breathing slowly and easily. Once your body is fully relaxed, you can follow with your mind. Thoughts and distractions will occur but, instead of fighting them, simply observe the movement of them in and through and past your quietly observing, detached mind, like water flowing over stones and weeds in a stream.

out breath
The letting go of the chest and diaphragm in a relaxed fashion as you breathe out, ideally followed by a small pause before the impulse to breathe in. This is simple way to calm the nervous system and find a natural rhythm to your breathing.

At this point you can choose to focus on a simple image in your mind's eye such as a single lit candle or, if you prefer, a scene which you find pleasant and relaxing such as lying on the beach watching the ripples on the shore, sitting in a meadow or by a river, lake or mountain side, or surveying a sunset or sunrise. It helps to choose the scene you will use in advance and to pick one that has happy memories for you. Stay there for about 20–30 minutes, and then slowly deepen your breath and open your eyes when you are ready to surface, fresh and rejuvenated.

Visualization sequence

If you have a pain that is intrusive during this sequence, you can choose a special visualization sequence to help reduce it. Once you are relaxed and have checked through your body, become familiar with the location of the pain and observe it in a detached way without the usual accompanying negative emotions. Find a shape that describes it. See if it has a colour and weight. Now choose one aspect, say red for its colour, and with each breath out watch the colour soften and lighten until it slowly changes into purple, then blue and green and yellow. If you only get as far as a soft pink, don't worry, that will do for now. Now focus on the shape of the pain, say a jagged shard, and see if with your relaxed breathing and gentle attention you can gradually smooth the shape into a more ball-like structure. Now watch the pain gradually shrink in size. Next focus on the weight. At first the pain may feel heavy, but with each breath it becomes lighter until eventually it is more like a cloud or mist. You now have a light yellow, puff of cloud that you can move with your breath slowly around your body and eventually down your legs and out through your feet – until it has gone. Don't worry if it bounces back – you are just practising a new skill that takes time to learn.

Ideally you should practise this daily for 20–30 minutes, and be patient as it may take a few weeks of regular practice before it comes easier and the benefits emerge.

Pathway options with optimal time course for back pain

M-S: Musculoskeletal, **'red flags'**: serious disease, **'yellow flags'**: psychosocial factors, **physical therapy** includes physiotherapy, osteopathy or chiropractic.

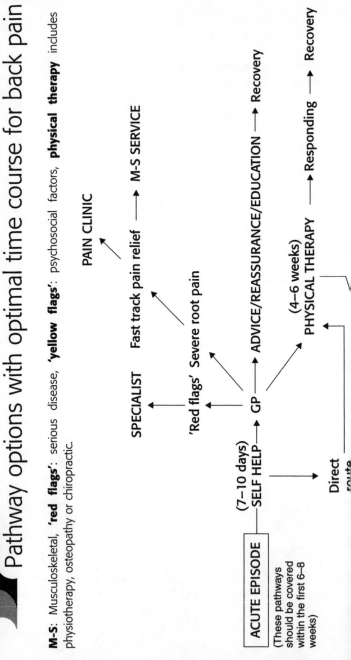

ACUTE EPISODE

(These pathways should be covered within the first 6–8 weeks)

(7–10 days)
SELF HELP

Direct route

GP → ADVICE/REASSURANCE/EDUCATION → Recovery

'Red flags' Severe root pain

SPECIALIST

Fast track pain relief → M-S SERVICE

PAIN CLINIC

(4–6 weeks)
PHYSICAL THERAPY → Responding → Recovery

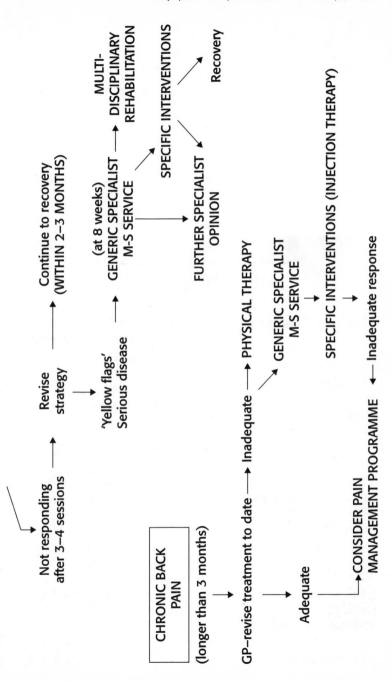

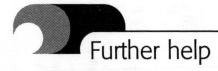

Further help

Useful addresses

Arthritis Care
18 Stephenson Way
London NW1 2HD
Helpline: 0800 289 170
www.arthritiscare.org.uk

Arthritis Research Campaign
Copeman House, St Mary's Court
St Mary's Gate, Chesterfield
Derbyshire S41 7TD
Tel: 01246 558 033
www.arc.org.uk

Back Care
16 Elmtree Road
Teddington
Middlesex TW11 8SE
Tel: 020 8977 5474
www.backpain.org

British Institute of Musculoskeletal Medicine
34 The Avenue
Watford
Hertfordshire WD17 4AH
Tel: 01923 220999
www.bimm.org.uk

General Chiropractic Council
344–354 Gray's Inn Road
London WC1X 8BP
Tel: 020 7713 5155
www.gcc-uk.org

General Osteopathic Council
176 Tower Bridge Road
London SE1 3LY
Tel: 020 7357 6655
www.osteopathy.org.uk

Manipulation Association of Chartered Physiotherapists

7 Warren Park Road
Hertford
SG14 3JA
Tel: 01922 589380
www.macp-online.co.uk

National Ankylosing Spondylitis Society

PO Box 179
Mayfield, East Sussex
TN20 6ZL
Tel: 01435 873527
www.nass.co.uk

National Osteoporosis Society

Camerton
Bath BA2 0PJ
Tel: 01761 471104
www.nos.org.uk

Pain Concern UK

PO Box13256 Haddington
East Lothian EH41 4YD
Tel: 01620 822572
www.painconcern.org.uk

Pain Society

21 Portland Place
London W1B 1PY
Tel: 020 7631 8870
www.painsociety.org

Society of Orthopaedic Medicine

39 Woodpecker Crescent
Burgess Hill
West Sussex RH15 9XY
Tel: 01444 241665
www.soc-ortho-med.org

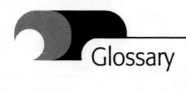

Glossary

Baseline levels
The level of activity or exercise that you can manage most days without increasing your pain intensity.

Catastrophizing
Thinking the worst, an extreme form of pessimistic thinking.

Cranium
The skull bones enclosing the brain.

CT scan
Computerized tomography scan.

Deconditioning
The loss of fitness resulting from prolonged rest.

Degenerating nucleus
The pulpy centre of the disc (nucleus) undergoing denaturing of its proteins due to enzyme action.

Demineralization
The leaching of minerals from your bones due to disuse.

Discs
The matrix of fibre and cartilage sandwiched between the vertebrae.

Disc protrusion
Protrusion of disc substance beyond the vertebral margins.

Discogenic pain
Pain arising from within the disc due to internal disruption of the annular layers of fibres.

Dorsal horn
The dorsal horn is the area of the spinal cord where sensory input from the periphery relays

with other nerves, some of which descend from the brain. It is the location of the 'pain gate mechanism'.

Downtime
Refers to time spent flat on your back resting during the day.

Epidemiology
The study of illness, disease and disorders in society.

Fear avoidance
A form of behaviour that some people develop as a result of anticipation of pain on movement, coupled with the belief that such pain is harmful and likely to make the condition worse.

Flexion curvature
Increased convexity of the spine.

Fluoroscopic control
The use of X-ray guidance to direct needles or other instruments accurately to the anatomical target.

Functional rehabilitation
An approach that focuses on function, rather than pain or damage, to return people to a more normal life.

Gait cycle
The pattern of movement of the legs when taking one complete step.

Gapping a joint
This describes the audible click or clunk accompanying a high velocity thrust type of manipulation indicating a full separation of the joint surfaces for a moment. It does not indicate a bone or disc being put back into place.

Herniation
Another term for disc prolapse.

Hypermobility
Refers to joints which have more than average flexibility due to ligamentous laxity.

Inhibitory and facilitatory pathways
Nerve tracts in the spinal cord that may either suppress or encourage the summation of pain impulses.

Innervation
Nerve supply.

Intervertebral foramen
The lateral canal through which the spinal nerve root emerges.

Lumbar instability
A controversial term which, in the context used here, refers only to the patient's subjective experience of their problem and the specialist's hypothetical explanation. It does not mean that there are any visible excessive movements of one vertebra on another.

Multifactorial	Indicates that the cause of a particular condition has many sources and influences.
Myofascial pain	Pain arising from the abnormal function of a muscle and its fascial covering.
Natural history	The course a disease or illness follows without interference from any form of medical intervention.
Neurogenic claudication	Pain and abnormal sensations arising from the nerves that are squeezed in a narrow spinal canal.
Neuropathic pain	Pain that arises from damaged or abnormally functioning nerve tissue.
Nociceptive pain	Pain that arises from stimulation of a pain receptor by a noxious event.
Osteochondritis	A disorder of the growth plate or ring of bone in adolescence, causing irregularity and alteration of vertebral shape.
Osteophytes	Outgrowths of bone resulting from remodelling and adaptation to stress and ageing.
Out breath	The letting go of the chest and diaphragm in a relaxed fashion as you breathe out, ideally followed by a small pause before the impulse to breathe in. This is a simple way to calm the nervous system and find a natural rhythm to your breathing.
Pacing	A strategy for maintaining a steady level of activity without the peaks that risk causing flare-ups of pain and troughs that result.
Palpatory skills	The ability to detect, purely by touch and passive movements, subtle changes in the soft tissues and joint play.
Pathology	Structural disease (as opposed to altered function which is reversible).
Post-traumatic stress disorder	A psychological state arising from a fright or shock when the person's survival has been threatened. This may follow any accident and bears no relation to the degree of injury actually sustained.
Radicular pain	Pain due to compression or irritation of a nerve root.

Red flags
These are the symptoms such as unexplained weight loss that may indicate more serious underlying disease and would prompt your doctor to investigate.

Simple back pain
This refers to 'non-specific' back pain. The pain arises from a mix of different tissues in the body and mechanical factors which are too complex for the expert to fathom.

Spinal fusion
An operation to fuse two vertebrae together using bone or metal implants.

Spinal stenosis
An excessive narrowing of the spinal canal.

Spondylo arthropathy
Inflammatory joint disease of the spine.

Spondylosis
The changes of the margins of the vertebra due to ageing.

Synovial fluid
Lubricating fluid that reduces friction in the joint.

Transitional vertebrae
An abnormal development of the vertebra structure and/or its joints.

Triage
A method first employed for military casualties in the Crimean war and now used to sort back pain into three useful categories requiring different approaches in management.

Trigger points
A 'knot' of hardened and contracted muscle that, when pressed or 'triggered' by various factors, refers to pain in a characteristic pattern.

Wear and tear
The preferred term for all the medical labels used to describe structural changes that occur with age and use (for example, spondylosis, degeneration, osteoarthritis).

Yellow flags
The term coined for the psychosocial factors (stress, depression, negative beliefs and fear of moving) that are risk factors for becoming chronically disabled.

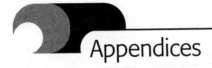

Appendices

Appendix 1: Lower back or leg pain
Appendix 2: Mid back pain
Appendix 3: Neck, shoulder or arm pain

The self-diagnosis flow charts on the following pages are designed to help you discover the possible cause of your back pain and your best course of action. However, it is important to remember that only a doctor can give a firm diagnosis of your sysmptoms.

Appendix 1: Lower back or leg pain

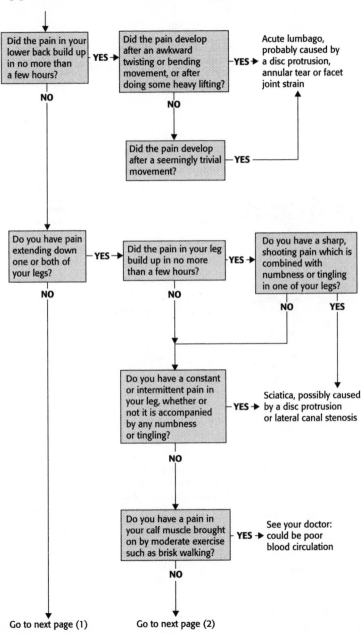

Did the pain in your lower back build up in no more than a few hours? — YES → **Did the pain develop after an awkward twisting or bending movement, or after doing some heavy lifting?** — YES → Acute lumbago, probably caused by a disc protrusion, annular tear or facet joint strain

NO

NO

Did the pain develop after a seemingly trivial movement? — YES →

Do you have pain extending down one or both of your legs? — YES → **Did the pain in your leg build up in no more than a few hours?** — YES → **Do you have a sharp, shooting pain which is combined with numbness or tingling in one of your legs?**

NO

NO

NO   YES

Do you have a constant or intermittent pain in your leg, whether or not it is accompanied by any numbness or tingling? — YES → Sciatica, possibly caused by a disc protrusion or lateral canal stenosis

NO

Do you have a pain in your calf muscle brought on by moderate exercise such as brisk walking? — YES → See your doctor: could be poor blood circulation

NO

Go to next page (1)   Go to next page (2)

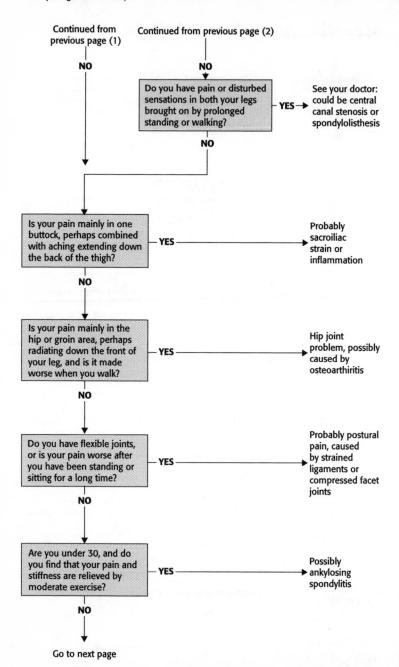

Continued from previous page (1)

Continued from previous page (2)

NO

NO

Do you have pain or disturbed sensations in both your legs brought on by prolonged standing or walking? — **YES** → See your doctor: could be central canal stenosis or spondylolisthesis

NO

Is your pain mainly in one buttock, perhaps combined with aching extending down the back of the thigh? — **YES** → Probably sacroiliac strain or inflammation

NO

Is your pain mainly in the hip or groin area, perhaps radiating down the front of your leg, and is it made worse when you walk? — **YES** → Hip joint problem, possibly caused by osteoarthiritis

NO

Do you have flexible joints, or is your pain worse after you have been standing or sitting for a long time? — **YES** → Probably postural pain, caused by strained ligaments or compressed facet joints

NO

Are you under 30, and do you find that your pain and stiffness are relieved by moderate exercise? — **YES** → Possibly ankylosing spondylitis

NO

Go to next page

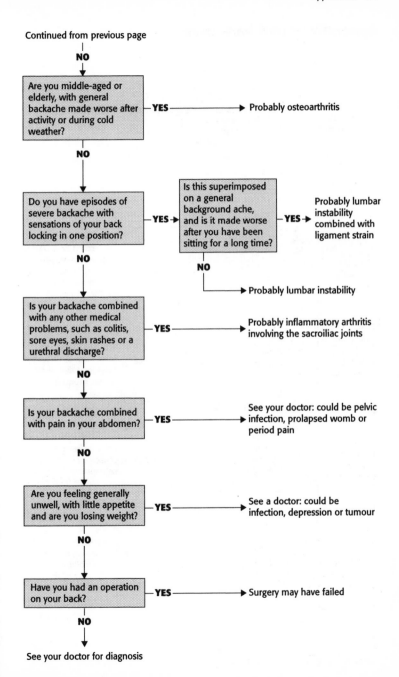

Continued from previous page

NO

Are you middle-aged or elderly, with general backache made worse after activity or during cold weather? — **YES** → Probably osteoarthritis

NO

Do you have episodes of severe backache with sensations of your back locking in one position? — **YES** → Is this superimposed on a general background ache, and is it made worse after you have been sitting for a long time? — **YES** → Probably lumbar instability combined with ligament strain

NO → Probably lumbar instability

NO

Is your backache combined with any other medical problems, such as colitis, sore eyes, skin rashes or a urethral discharge? — **YES** → Probably inflammatory arthritis involving the sacroiliac joints

NO

Is your backache combined with pain in your abdomen? — **YES** → See your doctor: could be pelvic infection, prolapsed womb or period pain

NO

Are you feeling generally unwell, with little appetite and are you losing weight? — **YES** → See a doctor: could be infection, depression or tumour

NO

Have you had an operation on your back? — **YES** → Surgery may have failed

NO

See your doctor for diagnosis

Appendix 2: Mid back pain

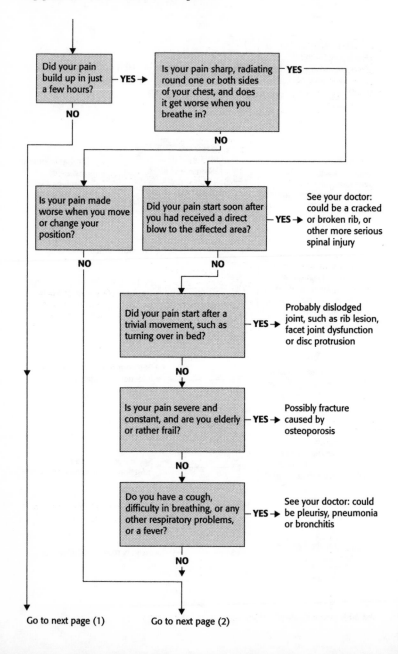

Did your pain build up in just a few hours? — **YES** → Is your pain sharp, radiating round one or both sides of your chest, and does it get worse when you breathe in? — **YES**

NO

NO

Is your pain made worse when you move or change your position?

Did your pain start soon after you had received a direct blow to the affected area? — **YES** → See your doctor: could be a cracked or broken rib, or other more serious spinal injury

NO

NO

Did your pain start after a trivial movement, such as turning over in bed? — **YES** → Probably dislodged joint, such as rib lesion, facet joint dysfunction or disc protrusion

NO

Is your pain severe and constant, and are you elderly or rather frail? — **YES** → Possibly fracture caused by osteoporosis

NO

Do you have a cough, difficulty in breathing, or any other respiratory problems, or a fever? — **YES** → See your doctor: could be pleurisy, pneumonia or bronchitis

NO

Go to next page (1)   Go to next page (2)

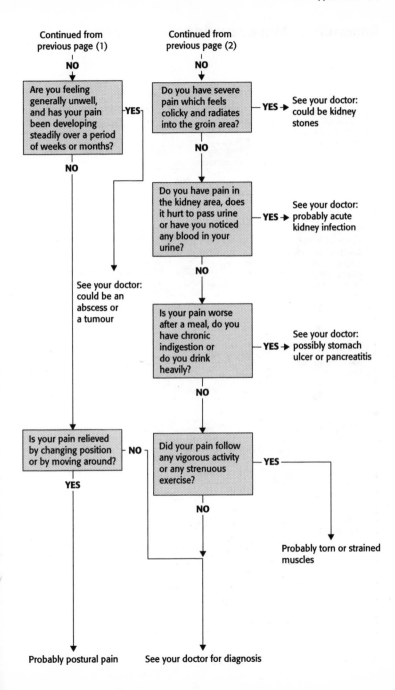

Continued from previous page (1)

NO

Are you feeling generally unwell, and has your pain been developing steadily over a period of weeks or months? —**YES**

NO

See your doctor: could be an abscess or a tumour

Is your pain relieved by changing position or by moving around? —**NO**

YES

Continued from previous page (2)

NO

Do you have severe pain which feels colicky and radiates into the groin area? —**YES**→ See your doctor: could be kidney stones

NO

Do you have pain in the kidney area, does it hurt to pass urine or have you noticed any blood in your urine? —**YES**→ See your doctor: probably acute kidney infection

NO

Is your pain worse after a meal, do you have chronic indigestion or do you drink heavily? —**YES**→ See your doctor: possibly stomach ulcer or pancreatitis

NO

Did your pain follow any vigorous activity or any strenuous exercise? —**YES**

NO

Probably torn or strained muscles

Probably postural pain

See your doctor for diagnosis

Appendix 3: Neck, shoulder or arm pain

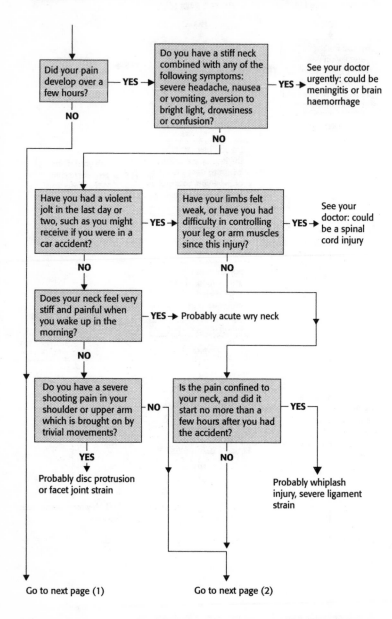

Did your pain develop over a few hours? — **YES** → Do you have a stiff neck combined with any of the following symptoms: severe headache, nausea or vomiting, aversion to bright light, drowsiness or confusion? — **YES** → See your doctor urgently: could be meningitis or brain haemorrhage

NO

NO

Have you had a violent jolt in the last day or two, such as you might receive if you were in a car accident? — **YES** → Have your limbs felt weak, or have you had difficulty in controlling your leg or arm muscles since this injury? — **YES** → See your doctor: could be a spinal cord injury

NO

NO

Does your neck feel very stiff and painful when you wake up in the morning? — **YES** → Probably acute wry neck

NO

Do you have a severe shooting pain in your shoulder or upper arm which is brought on by trivial movements? — **NO** → Is the pain confined to your neck, and did it start no more than a few hours after you had the accident? — **YES**

YES

NO

Probably disc protrusion or facet joint strain

Probably whiplash injury, severe ligament strain

Go to next page (1)

Go to next page (2)

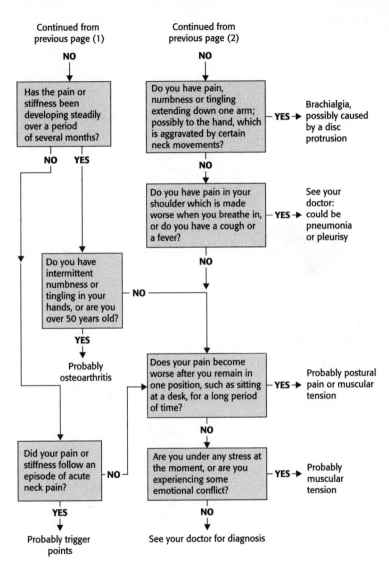

Continued from previous page (1)

NO

Has the pain or stiffness been developing steadily over a period of several months?

NO | **YES**

Do you have intermittent numbness or tingling in your hands, or are you over 50 years old?

— **NO** —

YES

Probably osteoarthritis

Did your pain or stiffness follow an episode of acute neck pain? — **NO** —

YES

Probably trigger points

Continued from previous page (2)

NO

Do you have pain, numbness or tingling extending down one arm; possibly to the hand, which is aggravated by certain neck movements? — **YES** → Brachialgia, possibly caused by a disc protrusion

NO

Do you have pain in your shoulder which is made worse when you breathe in, or do you have a cough or a fever? — **YES** → See your doctor: could be pneumonia or pleurisy

NO

Does your pain become worse after you remain in one position, such as sitting at a desk, for a long period of time? — **YES** → Probably postural pain or muscular tension

NO

Are you under any stress at the moment, or are you experiencing some emotional conflict? — **YES** → Probably muscular tension

NO

See your doctor for diagnosis

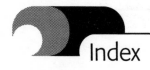

Index

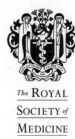

The ROYAL
SOCIETY of
MEDICINE

The Royal Society of Medicine (RSM) is an independent medical charity with a primary aim to provide continuing professional development for qualified medical and health-related professionals. The public benefits from health care professionals who have received high quality and relevant education from the RSM.

The Society celebrated its bicentenary in 2005. Each year it arranges and holds over 400 meetings for health care professionals across a wide range of medical subjects. In order to aid education and training further the Society also has the largest postgraduate medical library in Europe – based in central London together with online access to specialist databases. RSM Press, the Society's publishing arm, publishes books and journals principally aimed at the medical profession.

A number of conferences and events are held each year for the public as well as members of the Society. These include the successful 'Medicine and me' series, designed to bring together patients, their carers and the medical profession. In addition the RSM's Open and History of Medicine Sections arrange meetings on a regular basis which can be attended by the public.

In addition to the lectures and training provided by the RSM, members of the Society also have access to club facilities including accommodation and a restaurant. The conference and meeting facilities of the RSM were refurbished for their bicentenary and are available to the public for hire for meetings and seminars. In addition, Chandos House, a beautifully restored Georgian townhouse, designed by Robert Adam, is also now available to hire for training, receptions and weddings (as it has a civil wedding licence).

To find out more about the Royal Society of Medicine and the work it undertakes please visit www.rsm.ac.uk or call 020 7290 2991. For more information about RSM Press, please visit www.rsmpress.co.uk.